LOOK YOUNGER NOW

LOOK YOUNGER NOW

Fillers, Face Lifts and Everything in Between –

a 21st Century Guide

PATRICK M. FLAHARTY, M.D.

Patrick Flaharty, M.D.
Azul Cosmetic Surgery and Medical Spa
13470 Parker Commons Blvd
Suite 101
Fort Myers, FL 33912

www.AzulBeauty.com

ISBN: 978-1479317189
Printed in the United States of America
First Printing 2012

Cover design by Toten Creative
Page design and layout by Toten Creative
Author photograph by Nocera Photographic, Inc.

A NOTE TO READERS

Praise for Look Younger Now

"Dr. Flaharty has put together a comprehensive and easy read on a topic that the news, media and advertising has made complex. I am very impressed by the depth and scope of the book, and more so by the way in which the reader can connect to the material presented. The world of aesthetic medicine is ever-changing. A text like this, which covers the basics to the more complex, and is contemporary, concise and clear in structure, is an amazing and sorely needed aid and guide to anyone seeking cosmetic enhancement. I congratulate Dr. Flaharty for his efforts. Look Younger Now is a must-read for any patient considering a cosmetic procedure."

—Guy Massry, M.D.
Oculoplastic Surgeon
Beverly Hills, CA

"Look Younger Now is a must-read for those wanting to improve the look of their skin, or who are considering any kind of facial rejuvenation. It provides an educational, easy and comprehensive look at the wide range of options currently available to turn back the hands of time on the only face you've been given."

—Gina Birch
Journalist and Radio Personality
Southwest Florida

"Dr. Flaharty has written a well-rounded, honest and easy-to-understand guide to the aesthetic rejuvenation technologies available today. The patient stories are excellent, and really capture the different moods of why people have aesthetic services and the process they go through. This is a must-read for anyone who needs a no-nonsense education about what's available to them so, they too, can look younger."

—*Catherine Maley, MBA*
Author and Marketing Strategist
San Francisco, CA

"Look Younger Now is a well-written and easy-to-read primer for the woman or man considering "having something done." Dr. Flaharty demystifies the complexity of facial rejuvenation, empowering all of us who want to look younger. In fact, I was so motivated while reading the book, that I put it down, went to the phone and made an appointment!"

—*Marianne Swath*
patient for life
Ft. Myers, FL

"I certainly would like to commend Dr. Flaharty on this very thoughtful and comprehensive patient guide to facial rejuvenation. The explosion of options that have become available over the last ten years has resulted in a great deal of confusion for the patient consumer. Dr. Flaharty has done a wonderful job discussing not only the aging process, but putting in layman's terms all of the various options from the nonsurgical to surgical approaches. This guide will no doubt give clarity to anyone considering a facial rejuvenation procedure. Congratulations!"

—*Edwin F. Williams, III, M.D., FACS*
Williams Center for Plastic Surgery
Albany and New York City

Kudos for Dr. Patrick Flaharty

"I just want to thank you for helping me look years younger than I am. Many people are amazed when I tell them I am sixty-three years old. They think I'm in my forties."

—*Stephanie L.*

"Between your office and the surgical center it's like going to a five-star hotel and spa. Thank you very much!"

—*Tim G.*

"I didn't realize the results from fillers would be so great! Dr. Flaharty made me feel like I want to live again."

—*Dottie T.*

"Honestly, it was scary...who do I trust with the only face I have? I interviewed four plastic surgeons. I was getting discouraged with their attitude, approach and staff. Then I saw Dr. Flaharty. He was down to earth, dressed neatly and in good taste. I was received in the office with respect and honesty. He and his staff listened to me and looked me straight in the eyes. They were interested in me, what I wanted and what I wished for. I was put at ease; this was the surgeon for me. The result was dramatic! Dr. Flaharty pushed the sun up into the sky for me one last time and for that I will always be grateful."

—Phyllis S.

"I want to thank you and your staff for the excellent care. Everyone involved was highly professional and supportive throughout my surgery and post-operative period. Every step of the way, you and your staff told me what to expect, even though they knew I am a registered nurse. This meant a lot to me. I am so pleased with the results and would highly recommend you to all my friends. You and your staff have made my year special and refreshed! Thank you doesn't seem like it says enough about how wonderful you've made me feel about myself."

—Carol L.

"My face lift looks so natural that nobody—not even my friends—ever guessed! I am constantly being complimented on how youthful or great I look. Dr. Flaharty did a fabulous job, ensuring I would look natural, yet achieve the results I wanted."

—Lydia T.

To Kristen… amazing wife, loving mother, consummate professional and best friend.

Thank you for making my life truly extraordinary.

CONTENTS

About the Author

A board certified ophthalmologist and cosmetic surgeon, Patrick Flaharty M.D., has been in practice for more than twenty years, and has performed over 20,000 facial plastic and cosmetic procedures. He focuses exclusively on the face.

Having achieved a reputation as a premier facial cosmetic surgeon, Dr. Flaharty is sought after as a facial cosmetic surgery specialist, and has traveled throughout the world giving presentations on facial cosmetic surgery. He has spoken nationally at specialty meetings including the *Association of Ophthalmic Plastic and Reconstructive Surgeons* as an invited panelist, and as a course instructor at the *American Academy of Ophthalmology*. Dr. Flaharty has authored numerous scientific articles in medical journals including *Plastic and Reconstructive Surgery*®, *The American Journal of Cosmetic Surgery* and *Ophthalmic Plastic* and *Reconstructive Surgery.*

He is a graduate of the University of Michigan Medical School. After his residency at the prestigious Wills Eye Hospital in Philadelphia, Dr. Flaharty completed a two-year fellowship in ophthalmic and facial plastic surgery at the University of Utah. After several years of private practice, he completed a second two-year fellowship in facial cosmetic surgery in Orlando, Florida to further develop and refine his skills in the technical discipline of facial cosmetic surgery. He is a fellow of an elite group of less than 500 nationally trained eyelid surgeons (American Society of Ophthalmic Plastic and Reconstructive Surgeons) having successfully completed an approved fellowship as well as oral and written examinations. He is also a fellow of the American Academy of Cosmetic Surgeons, having completed an approved fellowship in facial cosmetic surgery and successfully completing the oral and written board examination in cosmetic surgery. Dr. Flaharty's twenty years of clinical experience—combined with his highly specialized training—make him uniquely qualified, and a true expert in facial cosmetic surgery.

He is a member of the American Academy of Cosmetic Surgeons, the American Academy of Ophthalmology, the American Society of Ophthalmic Plastic and Reconstructive Surgeons, the European Society of Ophthalmic Plastic and Reconstructive Surgeons, and the American Medical Association.

Since 1992, Dr. Flaharty has maintained an active medical practice in Southwest Florida. An avid supporter of education and the arts, he is an alumni representative on the Admissions Committee for the University of Michigan Medical School in Ann Arbor. Dr. Flaharty is passionate about sports and has served on the board of directors and is past president of the YMCA. He is a nationally licensed soccer coach, former president of the Florida Premier Soccer Club and an avid Miami Heat fan. In his leisure time, Dr. Flaharty enjoys tennis, running, and competing in triathlons. He recently competed in the Florida Iron Man, swimming 2.4 miles, biking 112 miles and then running a full marathon (26.2 miles.) He and his wife, Kristen, enjoy family time with their three daughters: Katie, Caroline and Kendall, and two golden retrievers.

Foreword

I am honored to write a foreword to Dr. Flaharty's excellent book, Look Younger Now. In my thirty-six years of training fellows in Oculoplastic and Facial Cosmetic Surgery, I have been privileged to mentor many of the best in the world, including Dr. Flaharty. I have learned as much from most of them as I have been able to teach. Dr. Flaharty has always been a gifted surgeon and a warm, caring physician. It is clear that he has continued to develop these qualities and they have become the cornerstone of his career. The years he spent with us at the University of Utah were memorable and enjoyable. He truly enjoyed surgery, often putting a face back together after trauma in the middle of the night. Following those stressful cases, Dr. Flaharty and I often biked, skied or hiked the beautiful Wasatch Mountains together— a great way to rebalance.

Over the past twenty years, eyelid and facial cosmetic procedures have exploded in numbers and evolved to safer, faster, more efficacious procedures with less downtime. With the large number of choices for cosmetic enhancement, choosing the right physician and procedure becomes complicated and confusing, and requires more patient knowledge today than ever before. Physicians are entering the cosmetic field of medical practice in large numbers, and are not always well-trained. Many have entered into the cosmetic arena due to the economic changes in medicine and the reduction of remuneration from the insurance industry. Combine the options for procedures, the number of doctors entering the field, the plethora of advertisements on the internet and elsewhere, and choices for consumers become even more risky and confusing. Dr. Flaharty shows that the best way to find a cosmetic surgeon is to evaluate training, experience, results, and prior patient or respected physician referrals.

Dr. Flaharty's book is an excellent overview of the cause, prevention, and treatment of facial aging. He consistently reinforces the message that patients want to look natural and more youthful rather than looking like they have had cosmetic surgery. He points out that one of the primary reasons for facial aging is the loss of tissue volume, and that an aging face is like a balloon slowly losing its air. The best skin rejuvenation procedures, use of injectables—including neurotoxins and fillers—and eyelid and facial cosmetic surgery procedures are presented in detail with their indications, but in an easy-to-read format. This book allows patients to key in on the problems that concern them, and then delve into potential solutions.

The patient stories comprise a wide array of surgical and nonsurgical procedures and age groups, including both men and women. These stories truly embody the reasons people decide to pursue cosmetic procedures and what they should expect to experience before, during and after the procedure. This glimpse into his practice is a testament to his expertise and results.

Dr. Flaharty's book is recommended for anyone considering facial cosmetic rejuvenation. He is to be congratulated for helping patients make more informed decisions regarding cosmetic procedures.

Richard L. Anderson, M.D., FACS
Medical Director, Center for Facial Appearances
Salt Lake City, UT
Former Professor and Chief,
Oculoplastic and Facial Cosmetic Surgery
University of Iowa and University of Utah

INTRODUCTION

· ·

Welcome to my world... and my passion:

Facial rejuvenation.

Would you like to look younger? Is there something about your appearance that bothers you? Have you ever looked in the mirror—or even just walked by a mirror—and wondered for a moment who was staring back at you? Have you ever said to yourself, "I just don't look like I feel?" or "What happened? I look tired and sad."

If your answer to any of these questions is yes, then get ready, because **this book may just change all that.**

Wrinkles, creases and folds, sagging facial features, crow's feet, lip lines, frown lines and brown spots may sneak up on us over a period of time... or they may seem to appear all at once. Either way, these changes in our faces (otherwise known as looking older!) are not welcomed with open arms by the majority of us. There was a time when "having something done" to look younger was a luxury afforded only by the wealthy. Thanks to new technologies and less invasive treatments, the world of facial rejuvenation and cosmetic enhancement is now available to the masses.

I love my work. I can't imagine anything more satisfying than sharing the excitement and happiness of a patient who looks in the mirror after a treatment or procedure. For the past two decades, I can truly say I've been excited to get up and go to work every day: I get to help people, to make them happier with themselves, and therefore, happier and more engaged with life. I wrote this book because I want to help you, too. If you've ever thought about "having some work done"— even if you've thought about it for only a minute —you know the idea of doing something to your face can be daunting. *Should I do it? What should I do? Is it safe? How long will it last? How much will it cost? Who should do it?* The "Twenty Questions Game" can result in paralysis.

I've written this book with *you* in mind. I want to answer your questions about what you can do to look younger. We'll discuss the aging process itself in chapter one. In chapter two, we'll talk about the major complaints and concerns I hear most often from my patients when it comes to their faces. I am sure you will relate to some of their stories. I've devoted chapter three to choosing the doctor who is right for you.

The second part of the book is devoted to the solutions that are available to you: from fillers to face lifts and everything in between. In chapter five, I'll reveal a secret to keeping a glow to your skin. Next are the quick fixes— such as BOTOX®[1] and fillers—available for busy people today. We'll cover those in chapters six through nine. I think you'll be surprised and excited to learn about the newest noninvasive lasers that can take years off your face. Did you know there's a way to tighten sagging skin without surgery? We'll discuss it in chapter ten. Surgery continues to remain "the gold standard" in facial rejuvenation for many men and women, and we'll take a look at surgical procedures in chapter eleven. By the way, this book is not just for women. Every treatment and procedure we discuss is available to both men and women. No longer is facial rejuvenation considered to be for women alone. The number of men taking advantage of Botox, fillers and surgical procedures is on the rise. In chapter twelve, I'll review some of the particulars for men only. Chapter thirteen is a "postscript on pricing."

When I decided to write this book, I asked some of my patients if they'd be willing to tell their stories. They all said yes. You'll find their stories, in their own words, woven throughout the book. I think you'll thoroughly enjoy reading accounts of real people—just like you—who thought about looking younger, and then took the bull by the horns and did something about it. I love Lynne's story: she and a group of girlfriends read Nora Ephron's book, *I Feel Bad About My Neck,* which ultimately led to a face

---

[1] *BOTOX® is the name of a product trademarked by its manufacturer, a company called Allergan. It is very common to see the word used generically. (This is no different than the word Kleenex being commonly used when referring to facial tissues.) The proper term is Botulinim Toxin Type A, which is a neurotoxin produced by three different companies.*

and neck lift for Lynne. You'll read about Ellie and her journey from skin cancer to skin care. Bill's account of an unfortunate surgery outcome, the result of choosing the wrong doctor, is compelling. I was thrilled to be able to help him.

Each story is unique. I did ask that each patient include whatever advice they would give to their best friend, if their best friend was thinking about facial rejuvenation. You get the benefit of advice from sixteen of my patients.

My philosophy: *facial rejuvenation must be very individualized.* As we surgeons go through our careers, we continue to learn. Our insights grow and change as new technologies and techniques make their way from the research lab into mainstream usage. It's easy to jump on the bandwagon thinking every patient needs this latest and greatest treatment or procedure. Having done nothing but facial surgery for twenty-two years and with so many tools available to us today, I believe I now have a much better sense of balance to my approach. I inform each patient of his or her options, and offer my opinion as to what would achieve the best result. Ultimately, it's a personal decision each patient must make. They still want to look like themselves, only younger and better. Sometimes patients need a little prodding to get the result they want, but in our office they are never pushed or sold.

Another part of my philosophy is *less is more.* Ultimately patients want the best possible result with the least amount of intervention and downtime. This must be balanced with the recognition that long-lasting, meaningful results can sometimes be achieved only through surgical procedures that require some downtime. (This is where the magic of the consultation comes into play.)

The last piece of my philosophy is to *offer facial rejuvenation in a caring, family-oriented practice.* We get to know our patients. We consider our patients to be part of our extended family and we're here for them. We see some of our patients monthly and many several times a year. Others we see every year or two. While we may see some patients only once, we do all we can to be supportive and caring—to make their time with us relaxing, enjoyable, and fun.

As I reflect on my patients and my practice, it seems both men and women come to the office initially for one of five reasons:

They...

1. feel young and vibrant but do not like what they see in the mirror.

2. have an upcoming event such as child's wedding or a class reunion.

3. feel the pressure in today's workplace to look younger.

4. have undergone a major life change such as divorce or the death of a spouse.

5. feel the need to make a life change.

Looking great knows no age. Taking steps to look younger is a personal decision each of us has to make. As you begin to consider facial rejuvenation, it is my hope that this book will be your guide, making your decision just a little bit easier. This book is not meant to be exhaustive. It is meant to provide an overview of the facial rejuvenation options available to you today: from fillers to face lifts and everything in between. It is meant to answer the questions I'm asked most frequently by my patients. Perhaps you'll have more questions when you finish the book. If so, please visit our website at www.azulbeauty.com or contact us to learn more. We are here to help you.

I'm delighted to be your guide. I invite you to turn the page and join me on a journey through the world of facial rejuvenation.

Patrick Flaharty, M.D.

ONE

....

INEVITABLE AND UNAVOIDABLE

All About Aging

Coco Chanel, the famous French fashion designer said, "Nature gives you the face you have at twenty. Life shapes the face you have at thirty. But at fifty you get the face you deserve." The problem is most of us aren't completely happy with the face we deserve. (More and more, this includes men as well as women.)

It's no secret that our perception of how we look influences not only how we feel about ourselves, but also our overall well-being. Studies—both in the United States and abroad—have proven this to be true. Think about a time when you were getting ready to head out the door, and you knew you looked great. You probably felt pretty terrific, too. Contrast that with a bad-hair day, or a time when you were running late and had to fly out of the house without your usual primping. It's possible you just didn't feel great about yourself that day. Here in the United States—as in many western countries—our view of a beautiful face has changed over the years. Like it or not, the flawless, seemingly forever-youthful face has become our standard of beauty for women. Hollywood, television programs, commercials, magazines and advertisements have all contributed to our concept of attractiveness in today's culture. While the approach of some is to celebrate age and accept all that comes with it, including a face with some lines and wrinkles, many approach aging with a sense of disappointment and a desire to turn back the clock.

Perhaps you're wondering where men fit into this picture on aging. For years, it has been not only socially acceptable for men to sport their gray hair and wrinkles, but expected. Today, more and more men are jumping on the anti-aging bandwagon: they're getting in shape, dying their hair, utilizing skin care and hair care products, eliminating unwanted hair, and yes…getting Botox, fillers and face lifts. In 2011, men had almost 800,000 cosmetic procedures, nine percent of the total. For the first time ever, face lifts were one of the top five procedures for men.[1] Men are no longer inhibited by a cultural expectation that says women are able to intervene on the aging process but men are not. That's a great thing for many men today.

HOW AND WHY DO OUR FACES AGE?

As we grow older, our faces reflect both our joys and our challenges in life. They also reflect our genes and our environment. Some of the factors that contribute to aging—such as fitness, nutrition and to a certain extent, our environment—are within our control. Other factors (genetics and gravity) are not within our control. As we age, our skin gets thinner and its elasticity decreases. Brown spots and other sun damage cause us to look older. At the same time, there are unavoidable changes happening under the surface: gravity pulls on our skin and muscles. When we're young, the fat in our faces is evenly distributed and abundant. (Think "baby face.") As we age, fat volume decreases and shifts, resulting in loose and sagging skin. The lower half of the face tends to gain fat. Jowls (drooping flesh under the lower jaw) form. Fat accumulates along the nasolabial fold (between the nose and creases of the mouth) and in the front of the neck. Fuller faces tend to remain youthful while thin faces do not age as gracefully.

Every day I hear complaints like Betty's, who felt her eyes made her look aged.

I Found My Plastic Surgeon By Accident

Betty

Age: 61

I'd wanted to have my eyes done for years, even when I was in my twenties. I had one lazy eye and as I aged, it got worse. When I turned fifty, I decided it was time for upper and lower eyelid surgery.

Excited at the thought of finally dealing with something that had bothered me for more than twenty years, I made an appointment for a consultation with a top-notch plastic surgeon. I ended up shocked and disappointed: he thought I might have ptosis. All I knew was that I had one eyelid that always drooped more than the other. I had never heard of ptosis. (It's a condition in which the eyelid droops abnormally, and the correction for that problem is different from a regular eyelid lift.) The plastic surgeon told me he did not do surgery for ptosis. He referred me to Dr. Flaharty, who is well-known as an eyelid surgeon. I decided that before I would make an appointment with Dr. Flaharty, I would go to my regular eye doctor. She agreed with the plastic surgeon that I had ptosis, and said the only person to do this surgery would be Dr. Flaharty.

Given that two top-notch doctors both referred me to Dr. Flaharty, I made an appointment with him. He agreed it was ptosis, but he was confident he could do surgery on both my upper and lower eyelids and fix my problem, so we scheduled the surgery. Then I went from being very excited to being scared to death. I'd never had anything done before and I was nervous the day of the surgery. Everyone at the surgery center was terrific and they put me at ease. Dr. Flaharty did both my upper and lower eyelids and it was everything I hoped for. It was pretty amazing.

That was in 2000 and I've been going to him ever since.

I was in the beauty business for twenty years: I owned a salon. When you're in the beauty business, you're especially conscious about looking your best. I wanted everything on my face to "match." My eyes looked really young—Dr. Flaharty did such an amazing job—but the rest of my face didn't, so I decided to get a brow lift and then a year later I had a mini-lift. I also had under-the-eye laser done. This was all within three years of having my eyelid surgery.

When Botox first came out, I said, "Sign me up." I've been doing it ever since. Now I go to Dr. Flaharty for maintenance (Botox and fillers) twice per year. Fillers last longer than Botox, so I get fillers once per year and Botox twice. One thing I really love about Dr. Flaharty is his "less is more" approach. I want to look better; I want to look refreshed, *but I don't want to look different. I've never made a secret of any of the work I've had done, so most people who know me, know I've had surgery. But... people who've never seen me before always assume I'm 10–15 years younger than I am.*

My advice to anyone who's considering getting some work done: it's really important to find a good doctor in your local area. Or, if you travel to get work done, I think it's important that you stay in the area while you heal. I say this because I have a girlfriend from New York who followed a doctor to Miami to have work done, and she had a bad experience.

Also, be sure to talk with several doctors and ask around in your circle of friends. Find someone you're 100 percent comfortable with, who has a great reputation, and who has a staff that's been with them for a long time. If you really can't afford to get work done, don't do it. If you're trying to save money, you're going in the wrong direction. Don't do it unless you can afford a great doctor. I would also tell anyone— male or female—don't wait! The younger you start, the better. We all spend a lot of years working and/or raising children. It's such a treat to do something for ourselves. Any time we look better, we feel better. Of course vanity steps in also. I'm a vain person in a comical way.

I have a funny story... I do ballroom dancing for a hobby. Debbie Reynolds is hosting the U.S. tour of the popular British show, "Senior Prom." They were looking for senior citizen ballroom dancers in our area, so I filled out an application and sent in my photo. I got a call back from a woman associated with the show. She thanked me for filling out an application, but she said, "You're tooooooo young!" Imagine how that made me feel.

A QUICK LESSON ON YOUR SKIN

Most of us don't give a lot of thought to our skin in general (other than the skin on our faces, and perhaps putting lotion on the rest of our body,) but in reality, skin is quite remarkable: the largest organ of the body, our skin is responsible for protecting us from dehydration, regulating body temperature, and shielding us from injury, disease and more.

The skin is essentially made up of two layers: the epidermis and the dermis. The epidermis is the top layer of the skin, the layer you see and feel. The epidermis itself is comprised of two layers: the outermost layer is called the stratum corneum; beneath the stratum corneum is the basal layer. The stratum corneum is composed of dead cells that have migrated from the basal layer. This migration of cells (cell renewal) happens over 15–30 days. As we age, the process of cell renewal slows down. The result is an accumulation of dead cells on the surface and a dry, scaly, lifeless appearance of the skin.

Beneath the epidermis is the dermis, which contains hair follicles, sweat glands, and nerve endings, along with collagen and elastin. Collagen is a protein that provides structure and support for your skin; it works hand in hand with elastin, which is a protein that keeps skin flexible.

The figure below shows how our skin changes as we age. Dead cells accumulate on the surface of the skin giving it a dry, scaly appearance while the critical proteins of collagen and elastin are gradually depleted from the deeper layers of the skin resulting in thinning, wrinkles, and loss of elasticity.

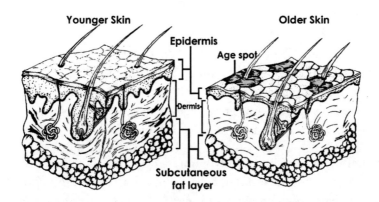

This illustration shows the anatomy of younger and older skin. Note the age spots, accumulation of dead skin cells, thinning of the epidermis, and the reduction of collagen bands present in the dermis of the older skin, compared with the younger skin.

TWO TYPES OF AGING

The aging process is a natural phenomenon, thus the skin ages naturally. This natural aging of the skin is call *intrinsic aging*. The skin also ages due to external factors—with the sun being the primary offender—and this is called *extrinsic aging*.

Intrinsic Aging

Here's the bad news about your skin: over time, collagen production slows, elastin loses its strength, dead skin cells do not shed as quickly, and new cells do not replenish as rapidly as they once did. This is a natural process and it happens to every one of us. It's called intrinsic aging, or chronological aging. The consequence of this natural aging process is loss of our skin's color, volume and elasticity. The result is dry skin, wrinkles, increased pore size, redness due to broken capillaries, and laxity. (Skin laxity essentially refers to the skin becoming looser.)

Our genes play a definitive role in the intrinsic aging process. We have zero control over the genes with which we're born. You've probably seen mothers and their daughters, or fathers and their sons, who have both grown older gracefully and who never seem to look their age. You may also have witnessed the opposite side of the coin: mothers and their daughters, as well as fathers and their sons, who appear to look older than their years. It's mostly in the genes.

Extrinsic Aging

Extrinsic aging results from exposure to external factors such as sun exposure, poor nutrition and sleep habits, smoking, extreme climates, pollution and stress. For the most part, these are factors over which we do have control. The consequences of extrinsic aging include deeper wrinkling, roughness, brown spots, a leathery look to the skin, and blotchy pigmentation.

The aging effect of the sun is called photo aging. Sun damage is the single biggest offender when it comes to facial aging. I can't stress this enough, so let me say it again: *sun damage to our skin is the single biggest offender when it comes to facial aging.* As much as eighty percent of the appearance of facial aging is due to sun exposure. In short, Ultraviolet radiation (UVR) from the sun causes skin damage. There are two types of UVR: the long-wave rays, called Ultraviolet A (or UVA for short) and the short-wave rays, called Ultraviolet B (or UVB.) Both UVA and UVB damage the skin and both need to be blocked or screened to reduce sun damage. It's the UVB rays, the short ones, that give you sunburn. The UVA rays, the longer rays, penetrate into the dermis, where they damage the collagen fibers. The result is skin damage.

WHAT ABOUT WRINKLES?

Wrinkles are lines that form in the skin. There are two types of facial wrinkles: dynamic and static. Wrinkles can be dynamic, static or a combination of the two.

Dynamic wrinkles form as a result of muscle motion—including the way we express ourselves—as well as from habitual movement, as is the case of vertical lip lines in smokers and crow's feet in tennis players who often squint in the sun. When our facial muscles contract, the skin over those muscles stretches to accommodate the muscles. When we're young, our skin bounces back after squinting, smiling or laughing. Eventually, however, our skin can no longer bounce back, and the dynamic wrinkles start to become more permanent, or static. The most common dynamic wrinkles are across the forehead, at the outer corners of your eyes (crow's feet) and between the eyebrows.

Static wrinkles are caused by gravity, the loss of fat and collagen, and the loss of the skin's elasticity. These types of wrinkles are visible regardless of the muscle action. They are always there, hence the term "static." Dynamic wrinkles eventually become static wrinkles. Some wrinkles are really more folds than lines, and may be dynamic or static. The deep lines that run from the nose to the sides of the mouth are called *nasolabial folds*. Lines that start at the corners of the mouth and go downward toward the jawline are called *marionette lines*. They form for three reasons: years of dynamic facial movements, static forces such as gravity, and chronological aging.

FACIAL DEFLATION

The single most important concept in facial aging is "facial deflation." As we age, the natural loss of fat—and to a lesser extent muscle and bone—leads to a loss of support for the skin and a sunken, hollow, sagging and drawn appearance to the face. (The gradual, progressive loss of fat in the face is called *global* fat loss.) Just as a deflated balloon loses it smooth, round exterior, a deflated face will flatten, sag, and wrinkle. This is one of the reasons fuller faces remain more youthful than thinner faces. Heavier people tend to age slower in the face.

BONE STRUCTURE

It's not only our skin that ages us. Changes in bone structure also contribute to making us look older. A study by physicians at the University of Rochester Medical Center[2] indicates that significant changes in facial bones occur as we get older, contributing to an aging appearance. The study noted that the angle of the jaw increases markedly with age, which results in a loss of definition of the lower border of the face. With the passing years, our cheekbones descend, offering less support. With the descending of our cheekbones, the eye sockets widen and become longer. This insidious loss of bone further contributes to volume loss and tissue sagging.

HOW WE AGE FROM DECADE TO DECADE

Some of us clearly recall the first time we looked in the mirror and noticed a line or two beginning to appear. One patient told me that when she looked in the mirror each day, she didn't really notice the signs of aging. Rather, it was when she walked past a mirror in a department store that she was taken aback. *Who was this person staring back at her?* She said, "I was absolutely shocked. I felt as though I had suddenly aged about ten years." Men often have a similar reaction, not necessarily because they have a few lines on their faces, but rather, it's the bags under their eyes or a receding hairline that gets their attention. Let's take a look at the aging of our faces, decade by decade.

Thirties

Many people notice signs of facial aging for the first time in their thirties. Expression lines such as crow's feet and laugh lines may begin to appear. There may be a trace of lines across the forehead and between the eyes. Upper eyelid skin can begin to droop. (The eyelids are the first area of the face that shows signs of aging: the skin is very thin and we blink twenty times a minute, which causes the skin to begin to wrinkle.) There may be some fine wrinkling at the outer corners of the lips. Skin may start to lose its glow.

Forties

In the forties, as we continue to lose facial collagen and elastin, more lines and wrinkles begin to appear. The areas that experience the most muscle movement are prone to more wrinkling: crow's feet around the eyes, smile lines around the mouth, and vertical lines around the lips. Lines across the forehead and between the eyes may become more pronounced. The compounding of time spent in the sun can be seen in uneven pigment and brown spots.

Fifties

Concerns during the forties become magnified for many in the fifties. The skin continues to lose its elasticity, causing deeper wrinkling. As fat padding in the face begins to diminish, cheeks may seem to drop, eyebrows may sag, eyelids may appear hooded, and jowls appear.

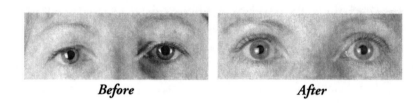

Before   *After*

Blepharoplasty (eyelid surgery) gives a rejuvenated appearance to the area around the eyes.

Sixties and Older

As we continue to lose facial volume (fat, muscle and underlying bone,) certain areas—such as the temples—begin to appear hollow. If you study the face of an older person, you'll see how the hollowing of the face contributes to aging as much as wrinkling does. We continue to lose elasticity resulting in sagging skin. Lines deepen in the forehead and between the eyes. Laxity and wrinkles lead to sagging of the neck tissue and the "wattle" appears in the front of the neck.

LIFE HABITS

Smoking, drinking, excessive sun exposure, poor nutrition and stress can all accelerate these aging changes. It behooves us to work at developing a balanced, healthy lifestyle to preserve not only our health and happiness, but also our looks.

THE PARADOX OF FITNESS

Thin athletic people tend to have minimal body fat. Although they may be in great physical condition, the lack of body fat may reveal itself in premature and accelerated facial aging such as hollow temples, sagging brows, dark circles under the eyes, flat cheeks, jowling, neck laxity and an overall gaunt appearance. Conversely, heavier individuals—although they may be overweight by traditional health standards—often retain more fat in the face preserving more of the youthful fullness and staving off many of the signs of facial deflation.

A FINAL WORD ON AGING

Aging is a part of life. We can't stop it, but we *can* take charge of it. Growing older is inevitable. Looking older is optional. We can age gracefully by caring for our skin, reducing our exposure to the extrinsic aging culprits, and taking advantage of new technologies, treatments and procedures in the world of facial rejuvenation. Turn the page to discover the complaints we hear most often in my practice. Some of them may sound familiar.

TWO

· · · · · · · ·

I Don't Like My _____!

Solutions for the modern man or woman

When it comes to the things men and women don't like about their aging faces, I think I've heard it all, from turkey necks to baggy eyelids to sun spots. Nothing surprises me anymore. When you look in the mirror, what bothers you? Perhaps it's the wrinkles that seemingly appeared out of nowhere. Maybe your skin has lost its glow. Is it the lines around your lips or the ones on your forehead? Perhaps it's your sagging neck. Is it the dark circles under your eyes or droopy eyelids? In the pages to follow, we'll look at the various problems and concerns, one at a time. Before we do that, I'd like to share Lynne's story with you. When Lynne came to the office for her consultation, the first thing I heard was, "I hate my neck!" I think you'll get a kick out of hearing how Lynne was ultimately inspired to have a face lift, after thinking about it for years.

Nora Ephron's Book Started it All

Lynne

Age: 59

In 2006, a group of girlfriends and I decided to read Nora Ephron's book, "I Feel Bad About My Neck." We gathered together one evening to discuss the book and after a few glasses of wine we all blurted out what we hated about our necks. Knowing I wasn't alone and that I had my friends for support, I finally had the courage to do something about it.

My neck was crepey and saggy, with deep lines: it made me look old. The trouble was— I didn't feel old! I had lots of energy; I'm a bit of a workaholic. I felt young, but I didn't look young. My motivation was simple: I wanted to look as youthful as I felt.

Having lived in Naples, Florida for more than twenty years, and being in the magazine business, I knew many cosmetic surgeons both professionally and socially. I quickly narrowed my search down to three doctors: two whom I knew both personally and professionally, and Dr. Flaharty, whom I knew only professionally. I made appointments with all three for consultations. For the first consult, a friend who had had a face lift herself went with me. She was very helpful and asked all the right questions. If you are lucky enough to have a friend with past cosmetic surgery experience to advise you and to even accompany you, I think it's much better than even bringing your spouse. Now I had an idea of what questions to ask and I was more prepared for the next two consults.

Each of the doctors whom I interviewed were equally competent, however, they all had different processes and fees, making it difficult to draw comparisons. Ultimately, I chose Dr. Flaharty for three reasons: first, he specializes in faces and that was important to me. Second, his physician assistant is incredible. (I thought so then and I still feel that way today. I want to call her the facial rejuvenation goddess or something like that.) She's genuine. She spent a lot of time with me. She shared numerous before and after photos with me, explaining each one, and carefully answered all my questions. She never once tried to sell me. My last reason for choosing Dr. Flaharty was the rest of his staff: they were caring and considerate. They worked with me to help me understand my options on the financial side. It was really the "Flaharty team" that sold me on going with Dr. Flaharty.

The possibility of having something done began back in 2006; however it wasn't until about six months before my surgery that I became serious. I was motivated to finally lose the extra twenty pounds I'd been carrying around and then I would schedule my surgery. (When you lose weight, you lose it in your face, so it's really important that you have your surgery while you're at your optimum weight.) It took me nearly six months to lose the weight. Because I was working full-time I knew the summer would be the best time to schedule my surgery. Once I had the three consults, I made up my mind within a few weeks and scheduled the surgery right away. I didn't have much time to be nervous or scared.

My daughter had just graduated as an RN, so she volunteered to fly to Florida and take care of me for three days. I ended up having a neck lift, face lift and brow lift. I think I was on an adrenaline rush after the surgery. The night of the surgery, I sat at home reading my Kindle. I had no pain at all. Two days later, I had my nails done. (I had only one very small bruise and I was able to cover it up with makeup.) During my recovery, I kept in regular contact with a few close personal friends via email. I sent them daily updates and daily photos. On day four, I was out riding my bike. Finally, on day seven, I came down a little from my adrenaline rush and I felt tired. However, I was back to work full-time in ten days. I was swollen for several months. They tell you about this in advance, but I didn't pay much attention to it. I did look a little different because of the swelling. Normally I have a square jaw, but after the surgery, I had a round jaw. It wasn't long before I looked like my old/new self again!

A few lessons learned: Don't expect your spouse to be totally supportive—that's what you have girlfriends for. Of course after the surgery my husband was much better. I don't think he liked the idea of my having elective surgery and that something might happen. I have a small regret: although all three surgeons did recommend a brow lift, I wish I had just had my upper eyelids done. Before, my forehead had no wrinkles and was tight…now I feel that the skin is much looser and my eyelids still need to be done.

In addition to the fact that I love the way I look, another great outcome of the surgery is that now I take much better care of my skin. I was a sun worshipper from a young age and had a lot of skin damage. I go to Dr. Flaharty's medical aesthetician for regular facials. I use all of their skin care products and makeup: I've used professional products all my life, but these are great, and extremely simple. I also bought a sonic cleaning brush for my skin and I use it with their cleanser. They have a wonderful sunscreen that has a little tint to it.

I'm always asking what else I can do to make my skin look better. I've had a little filler in my upper lip to fill out some wrinkles, but I don't really want to go the filler route. Right now I'm having fractional laser treatments to help get rid of those lines above my lip.

I have to laugh sometimes as I don't tell everyone that I've had a face lift. Most people know there's something different, but they don't know what it is. They just think I look good. My hair used to be short and I intentionally let it grow out to past my shoulders. A friend who had a face lift gave me this advice: change something about yourself before your surgery so people will notice that change— not your face lift.

My advice to others: do it for the right reason and do it for you, not for anyone else. Schedule at least three consultations. Be sure you have someone stay with you the night of your surgery and the next day. Best not to overdo it like I did—but with no pain and the adrenaline rush—it's tempting. If you need to lose weight, lose it before the surgery and keep it off for at least two months prior. If you plan to have a face lift, go to someone who specializes in faces alone.

One of my first purchases post-surgery was a beautiful twelve-inch gold necklace. I no longer feel bad about my neck. In fact, I love my neck!

We see Lynne at Azul on a regular basis and she's an inspiration to us all. Now let's take a look at all the problems and concerns I hear about every day. Just like Lynne, the words I hear most often are "I don't like my _____!"

DYNAMIC WRINKLES

As we said in chapter one, dynamic wrinkles are the lines you see when the face is moving: forehead lines, frown lines, laugh lines and crow's feet. They're formed as the result of repeated facial expression, and may create an appearance of stress, tension or fatigue. Dynamic wrinkles generally respond well to Botox.

Forehead wrinkles – or lines across the forehead. Some would say forehead lines are more acceptable in men than in women. Men tend to look distinguished with lines in their brow, while women think they just look old.

Treatment: Botox or a brow lift

Crow's feet – also called "laugh lines," these are the wrinkles that form at the outside corners of the eyes. The only way to avoid crow's feet is to never squint, laugh, or smile.

Treatment: Botox, chemical peel, laser peel

Frown lines – are those vertical lines between the eyebrows. Severe frown lines can make a person look angry or stern.

Treatment: Botox for fine lines, Botox and fillers for deeper lines

STATIC WRINKLES

Static wrinkles persist even when there is no muscle tension. In other words, any wrinkle that does not disappear when the face is at rest is a static wrinkle. Dynamic wrinkles will become static wrinkles over time. Static wrinkles can also result from sun damage combined with years of muscle contraction. Static wrinkles may be treated with fillers, medical-grade peels, lasers, and lifting procedures.

Lip lines – are sometimes called smokers' lines, but you don't have to smoke to get lip lines. They are the result of talking, laughing, eating and expressing ourselves. Women have a particular concern about these lines because lipstick tends to "bleed" into the lip lines.

Treatments: Botox, fillers, dermabrasion, lasers

Overall facial lines – are most often caused from sun damage and the natural aging process.

Treatments: microdermabrasion, skin care with a product containing Retin-A, lasers, lifting procedures

DEEP LINES OR FOLDS

As we age, the combination of the constant pull of our facial muscles combined with loss of volume and elasticity can result in deep lines or folds. The two prominent areas for these folds are both around the mouth: the nasolabial folds and the marionette lines. Deep lines or folds may be treated with fillers or surgery.

Nasolabial folds – sometimes called smile lines, these deep lines run from each side of the nose to the corners of the mouth.

Treatment: fillers, face lift, fat transfer

Marionette lines – or frown lines, start at the corners of the mouth and extend downwards. They make us look as though we're frowning.

Treatment: fillers, face lift, fat transfer

SAGGING AND BAGGING (SKIN LAXITY)

A natural consequence of aging is that our skin loses its elasticity. Gravity, sun damage and loss of collagen and elastin all have a role in the sagging and bagging we see in the mirror, as does the loss of underlying fat in our faces. As we get older, the skin just doesn't bounce back as it once did. The treatment for sagging and bagging depends on the severity of the problem and may include a skin-tightening procedure or surgery.

Sagging neck – sometimes referred to as a turkey neck or wattle. There's a general tendency to take care of our faces and neglect our necks. Proper skin care for the neck area is just as important as it is for the face.

Treatment: face and neck lift, neck liposuction, Ultherapy®

Jowls – is the term for loose skin and fat under the lower jaw. Jowls are caused from loss of facial volume, loss of elasticity with skin stretching, and gravity pulling the skin and fat downward. Some of my patients refer to their jowls as a "saggy jawline."

Treatment: face and neck lift, Ultherapy

Crepey skin – refers to fine, wrinkled skin which has lost its smooth surface. Crepey skin is caused from loss of collagen and sun damage. The skin takes on a dry, wrinkled, lifeless appearance as a result.

Treatment: skin care with Retin-A, micropeels, chemical peels, laser peels

Drooping eyelids – Both our upper and lower eyelids can droop as we grow older. The upper eyelid sags, sometimes to the point of causing impaired vision. Women complain, "My eye shadow doesn't even show anymore." Sagging upper eyelids is often the first thing to bother someone; this was the case for Shannon, a figure competitor. (You'll read her story in chapter twelve.)

Treatment: eyelid surgery, Botox, Ultherapy.

DARK CIRCLES AND THE TIRED APPEARANCE

Facial volume loss is inevitable and is the result of the decreasing facial fat, muscle, and bone, which leads to the sagging of facial tissue. As we age, our cheek bones seem to disappear. Our faces begin to appear less round than the full face of youth. Our lips get thinner. Treatments for these concerns include fillers, fat transfer and the face lift.

Dark circles – a sunken look under the eyes is from a loss of volume—a decrease in the amount of fat and supportive tissue. Hollowing under the eyes can make you appear very tired.

Treatment: fillers, fat transfer

Thinning lips – lips thin out and go from being bow-shaped and full to skinny and shapeless. Full lips are a sign of youth and vitality. They encourage us to laugh and smile. Thin lips look old and lifeless and can lead to frown lines at the corners of the mouth.

Treatment: fillers

Flat, sunken cheeks – a young face has fullness and roundness in the cheeks. As we lose soft tissue and bone, our cheeks lose their prominence, resulting in a hollow, flat look to the cheeks and multiple contours through the cheek area.

Treatment: fillers, fat transfer, face lift

SKIN PROBLEMS

Many of our patients start as skin-care patients. They come to us with complaints of brown spots, redness in their skin, large pores, uneven skin tone, and more. These problems are largely the result of sun damage. Treatments for these problems include skin care, peels, lasers and fillers.

Brown spots – sometimes called sun spots or age spots, are small areas of hyperpigmentation. They are usually the result of too much sun exposure. Genetics may also play a part.

Treatments: skin care, peels, lasers

Acne/acne scarring – acne can occur at any age, starting in the teenage years. Hormonal changes in perimenopause and menopause are known to provoke pimples, so it's not uncommon for our female patients in their forties and fifties to experience acne. As one patient said to me, "It's just not fair. I didn't have acne as a teenager. Now I have acne and wrinkles at the same time."

Treatment: skin care, peels, lasers, fillers

Large pores – in most cases, you can blame your parents for your large pores. Genetics plays a major role in the size of your pores. Large pores aren't easy to treat, though there are a number of solutions for reducing the appearance of large pores.

Treatment: skin care, lasers

Melasma – a patchy brown or tan discoloration on the face, melasma is seen mostly in women. The exact cause isn't known. Melasma is difficult to cure but it can be managed with specific treatments.

Treatment: skin care, lasers

Redness in the skin – facial skin that appears red is usually the result of broken capillaries, or Rosacea—a chronic, inflammatory skin condition.

Treatment: skin care, lasers

The normal aging process, coupled with lifestyle choices, can cause us to gradually lose our youthful glow. For some, self-image can deflate when their skin begins to lose its luster. My role is to educate patients on the myriad of solutions available today to help combat aging and thus improve the way women and men view themselves as they age. Like anything else in life, where there is knowledge, there is power, and facial rejuvenation certainly is no different. By arming patients with good information, they are able to make educated decisions about how to look and feel their very best—at any age. In the next chapter, I'll begin to help you move through some of the steps toward making the right choices for you.

THREE

· · · · · · · · · · · ·

Do Your Homework

Choosing the right doctor will make a difference

A t the risk of stating the obvious, selecting a highly qualified, experienced doctor is a significant decision and perhaps the single most important factor in ensuring the success of any facial rejuvenation procedure. For some, making the decision to enter the world of facial rejuvenation is an easy one; others ruminate over the thought of picking up the telephone to schedule a consultation. I've heard plenty of stories about individuals who make the decision to have a procedure, only to proceed at breakneck speed, selecting the wrong doctor for the wrong reasons in their fury to forge ahead with their plans for facial rejuvenation. Please take time to do your homework. We've all seen friends or television personalities, heard stories or seen photos, of post-surgery faces that appear to have been caught in a hurricane or lips inflated to cartoon-character proportions. Simply put, they look unnatural, and nobody wants that, neither the patient nor the doctor. New patients are not hesitant to share their previous, unpleasant experiences with me and my staff: one patient told us she never even saw her surgeon before she went under anesthesia. When there were complications after the surgery, the surgeon was unwilling to deal with them. The American Board of Cosmetic Surgery advises choosing a doctor based on their education, training, experience and proven competence with respect to the specific procedure you are considering. Take the time to do your research, including meeting with potential doctors, to ensure you make the best choice of doctor for you.

HOW TO FIND A DOCTOR

Doctors develop their reputations based on results. Therefore, a word-of-mouth referral is a great way to find a doctor. Do you have friends who've "had work done" and love the result? If so, talk with them about their experience and get the name of their doctor. Inquire about a doctor's reputation in your community. Your primary care physician, dermatologist, gynecologist, or ophthalmologist may be able to recommend a doctor for facial rejuvenation. Ask your doctor where he would send his own family members. Take these recommendations seriously, as they are one of the best unbiased sources of information.

In some parts of the country—California, New York and Florida in particular—there's a great deal of competition when it comes to face lifts, injectables such as the neurotoxins or fillers, etc. This is an advantage for you. If you live in these areas, don't be surprised to see doctors advertising in newspapers, magazines and on television. These types of promotions provide you more exposure to doctors and the services they offer. Many doctors conduct complimentary seminars. Attending such an event is a great way to get a feel for the doctor, an overview of the procedures offered at his or her office, and in many cases to see the office and samples of the doctor's work first hand, with no commitment.

DO YOUR HOMEWORK

Legally, not every facial rejuvenation procedure must be performed by a doctor. For example, in the state of Florida, Advanced Registered Nurse Practitioners (ARNPs) and Physician Assistants (PAs) can administer injectables and perform laser procedures, working under the protocol established by the doctor. No other healthcare professionals though, including RNs or LPNs, can perform these services. In some states, nurses are actively injecting neurotoxins and fillers; licensed cosmetologists and aestheticians are performing laser hair removal and photo rejuvenation with intense pulsed light devices. However, this is not the practice in Florida.[3] The key to success with paramedical professionals administering these treatments lies in the level of training they've had, and their relationship with the doctor with whom they work. If you are seeing a nurse for these treatments, look for one who is working with a single doctor, not a "nurse for hire" who floats to the offices of various doctors. If you want to come back for any reason, you want to know that the nurse who performed your injections—or the doctor—will be in the office to see you.

In each state, the Board of Medicine governs doctors, and the Board of Nursing governs nurses; these boards control who is allowed to perform various procedures. It's your job to learn about the regulations in your state. Buyers beware: we've all heard "Botox Party" horror stories, and other bad outcomes from facial rejuvenation procedures. If something sounds too good to be true, it probably is. I'm sometimes asked why different types of medical doctors—including dentists, gynecologists and internists—are injecting the neurotoxins (such as Botox) and fillers. The answer is twofold: first, they are permitted to do so by the Board of Medicine in their state and second, these procedures can add to the profitability of their practices. While I have nothing against my colleagues who practice different types of medicine, my suggestion is to consult with a facial cosmetic surgeon.

Those who live and breathe faces—day in and day out—are the ones most likely to give you, the patient, your best result. You wouldn't have a dentist deliver your baby, would you? We sometimes have prospective patients call to inquire about prices for the different injectables and upon learning our fees, they suggest our prices are too high. Upon further discussion, we discover they previously had injections by a dentist who charged less, yet the patients weren't happy with the result. These treatments have become a commodity in today's world. The experience and level of relevant education of the practitioner who administers these products is critical in achieving the result you desire. Remember...there is no substitute for experience. Here's a story from one of my patients who learned the hard way that doing your homework is absolutely crucial.

I Had Resigned Myself to Living the Rest of My Life With a Terrible Plastic Surgery Outcome

Bill

Age: 61

Seven years ago I had a face lift. I'm in a very high-stress business that had taken its toll on me. I felt as though I looked way older than my years and I wanted to do something about it. I started asking around and was referred by more than one person to the doctor who ultimately did my face lift. I knew several people who were happy with her. She even repaired a cleft palate for the son of one of my friends. In fact, she does a lot of pro bono work for kids with cleft palates in third world countries.

While I was happy with the face lift itself, I had some serious complications: my neck would not stop draining and I had drooping under my chin. In addition, my lower eyelids drooped to the point where you could see the red capillaries all the time. It was awful. After about six months, when the problems persisted, I went to another plastic surgeon for a consultation. He said he couldn't help me. I resigned myself to living with it for the rest of my life.

I had found my plastic surgeon by word of mouth, but I should have done more research on her. I later learned that she had been banned from doing surgery at the local hospital because she'd done so many surgeries with bad outcomes.

This past winter, I was visiting my sister in Ft. Myers, Florida. I went to get a haircut and as the guy was cutting my hair, it dawned on me that he looked great, so...I asked him if he'd had work done. He had. This guy was probably sixty-two or sixty-three, but he looked like he was in his forties. He wasn't overly done. He just looked terrific. He referred me to Dr. Flaharty (who had done his face lift) so I timidly made an appointment for a consultation.

When I walked into Dr. Flaharty's office, it was comforting to see a professional staff as opposed to a one-man operation. Just talking with Dr. Flaharty and reliving my surgery was nerve-wracking. Of course I was hesitant to do a second surgery, but I also very much wanted to have my problems fixed. My eyes were a constant problem. I told Dr. Flaharty that I had a horrible recovery after my surgery: pain, swelling, tubes...and I was so black and blue. He assured me none of those things would be the case if I did a second surgery with him. I decided to go for it.

I was terrified when I went in for the second surgery with Dr. Flaharty. I was jumping out of my skin. As soon as I arrived at the surgery center, they gave me some "calm-down" drugs because they knew how nervous I was. The head nurse gave me the complete rundown, and then they wrapped me up and made me very comfortable. Next, the *anesthesiologist came in to talk with me. (My first doctor didn't even have an anesthesiologist.) After we talked, he gave me something intravenously to help calm me even more.*

Dr. Flaharty fixed everything: he repaired my eyes using skin grafts. I also had huge lumps and scars behind my ears. He fixed all that. The first surgeon didn't do my neck in the back, so Dr. Flaharty repaired my neck.

I'm thrilled with the result. You can probably guess my advice to others: whatever you do, be sure to do your homework when you're looking for a doctor to work on your face. I didn't do any research on the Internet and I should have.

PROCEDURE-SPECIFIC EXPERIENCE

The explosion in cosmetic procedures in recent years has resulted in growing competition among physicians. When considering facial rejuvenation, education, training, experience, and proven competence with the procedure you are considering are extremely important criteria in selecting the right surgeon. Board certification is often touted as important criteria in distinguishing one doctor from another. It is certainly an important first step on the path to becoming a cosmetic surgeon, but unfortunately, board certification does not necessarily connote competence—let alone expertise— in any given procedure. The truth is, the world of cosmetic surgery is evolving very rapidly and is shared by physicians from multiple disciplines including plastic surgery, facial plastic surgery, oculoplastic surgery, dermatology, and maxillofacial plastic surgery. In recent years, even physicians from gynecology, internal medicine, and family practice have incorporated cosmetic procedures into their practices.

There is no substitute for experience. When you are considering a cosmetic procedure, you need to know the physician's competence with the specific procedure: How long has the doctor been performing the procedure? How many procedures do they do in a week, a month, or a year? Ask to speak with patients who have had the same procedure. Check the online reputation of the doctor and practice. Generally people build successful cosmetic practices by specializing in a specific area and delivering exceptional results. Good results lead to happy patients and new referrals. When choosing a physician, do your homework.

COSMETIC SURGERY VERSUS PLASTIC SURGERY

Cosmetic surgery and plastic surgery are not the same. *Cosmetic* surgery is elective surgery with the goal of a pleasing aesthetic outcome. The historical focus of *plastic* surgery is reconstruction or repair, such as breast reconstruction surgery after a mastectomy, skin cancer surgery, or the repair of a birth defect such as a cleft palate. A cosmetic surgeon is principally trained in another discipline such as plastic surgery, facial plastic surgery, oculoplastic surgery or maxillofacial plastic surgery and has chosen to focus on cosmetic procedures. Although most cosmetic surgeons are first trained as plastic surgeons, not all plastic surgeons are cosmetic surgeons. A plastic surgeon doesn't necessarily focus on cosmetic surgery, and may do an array of procedures on all parts of the body. This is important when choosing a surgeon because training alone does not tell you the specific focus of the practice or how much experience a surgeon has with a specific cosmetic procedure. In general, your interests are best served in the hands of a busy specialist. Again, do your homework.

YOUR CONSULTATION

Having done your homework and narrowed the field of potential doctors, your next step is to schedule at least one, and preferably two or three, consultations. Some doctors charge for a consultation; others do not. The cost for a consultation can range from $50–$250 or more. Many doctors credit the cost of the consultation toward any procedure performed. Go to your consultation well-prepared. You may even consider bringing a list of questions; I have provided some sample questions below to help you comprise one.

During your consultation, the doctor will ask you about your specific concerns. Using his education, training and expertise, he will advise you on what you can improve, and the specific procedure(s) to accomplish your goals. In the initial patient consultation, I always address the patient's concerns first. Once I understand the patient's goals, I examine the entire face in detail including the skin, fat, muscles, bones, and overall shape and tone of the face. This leads to what I call a "facial profile," which is essentially a list of the patient's surgical and nonsurgical options. Those options are then combined with the patient's concerns, resulting in a detailed summary of the best options for that patient. In addition to addressing the patient's immediate concerns, I always offer other options that would help the patient look better, feel better, and enjoy his or her appearance more. Sometimes there is more than one solution to a problem, in which case I will present all of the options. Some patients come to me having no idea of the procedure that will resolve their concerns; others may be considering a specific procedure, only to learn they will benefit more from a different procedure.

As with all professional relationships, you must feel completely comfortable with the doctor you choose to perform a procedure on your face. Do not be afraid to query the doctor or his staff. You may think your question is odd, but I doubt anyone will be surprised by any question you pose. Believe me, we've heard it all. You'll want to know how often the doctor has performed a specific cosmetic procedure, and any downside to the procedure. Ask to see "before and after" photos of the doctor's own patients who have had the procedure you're considering. Of course, you'll want to know the cost of your potential procedure. Other questions might include...

- the doctor's education and training including medical school, residency and fellowships

- how long they have practiced in the current community

- information about the facility if surgery is to be performed

- type of anesthesia (if it will be used) and who will administer it

- any potential risks or side effects

- any preparation you need to do before the procedure

- anticipated recovery time

- length of the procedure

- level of pain that might be involved

- any post-procedure care you will need to provide for yourself

- how long before you can resume your normal activities

- After your consultation, ask yourself some questions:

- Was I comfortable with the surgeon?

- Did he or she answer all my questions?

- Did the staff make me feel welcome and comfortable?

- Would I send a friend here?

Choosing the right doctor can make all the difference between a good and an unfortunate experience. Take the time you need to make your decision. Please do not base your choice of a doctor on cost alone; be sure your surgeon is well-trained and highly-experienced. In my practice, we have numerous patients who have become "patients for life." Our patient, Ann, has become one of those patients for life, even though she doesn't live in Florida year-round.

I Went From Skin Care to Surgery

Ann

Age: 51

I've had problematic skin ever since our kids were born. I developed acne and along with it, the resulting pock marks. I hadn't felt good about my skin in years. Nine years ago, we were on vacation in Ft. Myers Beach. I was reading the paper and saw an ad for a plastic surgeon's office that offered specialized skin care, so I made an appointment. It was Dr. Flaharty's office. I went for my consultation and they put me on a skin care program that really made a difference. I'm still with them; I'm still using their products. Even though I'm nine years older, my skin looks so much better today than it did nine years ago. My skin is so much nicer, more clear, firmer and toned.

At Dr. Flaharty's office, they have a "less is better" philosophy when it comes to skin care and I really like that. The products are simple: in the morning, I use a glycolic cleanser, an oil-free hydrating fluid, eye serum and sunscreen, SPF 30. I also use their makeup, which is Jane Iredale. I love the foundation. At night, I have a simple routine with the cleanser and the same hydration I use in the morning. That's it!

We used to visit Florida every year for vacation. Now we have a place there and that's where we spend our winters. After about two years on the skin care products, I started to get Botox and fillers. No one at Dr. Flaharty's office ever pushed me to do it. I knew everyone in the office by that time and I knew Dr. Flaharty's work. I was very comfortable with him and just decided I wanted to do something more than skin care.

Then one day I was looking in the mirror and realized I no longer looked vibrant. I looked tired. I had a consultation with Dr. Flaharty and we decided on doing my lower eyelids and TCA Peels around my eyes. A year and a half later, I did my upper eyelids. Five years ago, I had liposuction under my chin.

I'm diligent with taking care of my skin. In addition to using the products, I now go for monthly facials when I'm in Florida. I still have some problems with clogged pores, so I get skin peels with the aesthetician every four months. Sometimes I get microdermabrasion. A few years ago, I started photo rejuvenation laser treatments with Dr. Flaharty's physician assistant. Now I have touch ups once each year. I can't get to Florida as often as I'd like to in the summer, but I won't go to anyone else. If I can't get to Florida, I live without it until I can get there.

Last winter, I did an S-lift. It's a mini face lift for anyone not ready for a complete face lift. I'm always a little nervous about being put to sleep, but I completely trust Dr. Flaharty. When you do things to your body, you need someone you can trust. My husband took me to the surgery center. I was there for about four hours. I took one pain pill right after the surgery and then just Ibuprofen after that. I had no black and blues at all. It did take a full year before the numb feeling around my ears went away.

People always tell me I look great. The skin care makes all the difference. I keep up with the laser light treatments and the peels. Of course the fillers and Botox help, but my main thing is the skin care. People tell me my skin glows. In fact, Dr. Flaharty's office has taken care of our youngest son and our daughter-in-law, both for skin care.

The biggest piece of advice I can give anyone is to do your homework before you decide on a medical aesthetician or a doctor who will do anything to your face.

While some of our patients may have started coming to Azul for skin care or perhaps fillers, they now come to the office on a regular basis. Others began with a face lift and subsequently take advantage of all our other services to stay looking their best. In choosing your doctor, consider the fact that you, too, may be choosing "a cosmetic surgeon for life."

FOUR

· · · · · · · · · ·

THE PYRAMID OF SOLUTIONS

A primer on facial rejuvenation

Never have there been more treatment options available in the world of facial rejuvenation than there are today. Thanks to new technology, materials and techniques, facial rejuvenation procedures are wildly popular, growing more so by the day. The pyramid of rejuvenation is a concept I've used for years in my seminars to categorize facial rejuvenation treatments based on their level of invasiveness. It is important to note that although the categories in the pyramid remain relevant over time, the actual products and procedures moving in and out of the pyramid are constantly changing as new, more effective products and procedures replace older, obsolete techniques. So, although the framework stays the same, the content of the pyramid is constantly changing.

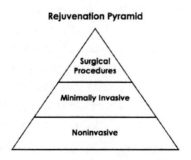

The base of the pyramid contains all the noninvasive treatments and technologies available to patients. Noninvasive treatments are those that do not require injections or surgery: skin care, (specifically micropeels, microdermabrasion, dermaplaning and topical cosmeceuticals,) as well as the exploding field of noninvasive lasers and technologies to rejuvenate, tighten, and lift the skin. This category has been one of the fastest growing and exciting areas in the arena of cosmetic facial rejuvenation. The number of noninvasive procedures and technologies that can achieve dramatic rejuvenation of the face and neck is amazing. Staying abreast of the latest and greatest products and procedures in this broad base of the pyramid is a full-time job. A very important part of our practice is to screen and select the best products and procedures to offer our patients.

The first of the noninvasive treatments is skin care. According to *Milady's Standard Textbook for Professional Aestheticians*, by Joel Gerson, "A healthy skin is slightly moist, soft, flexible, possesses a slightly acid reaction; and is free from any disease or disorder."[4] Healthy skin is a great place to begin when it comes to facial rejuvenation. All other procedures and treatments will be enhanced by healthy, glowing skin.

Good skin care starts in the hands of a good aesthetician who conducts a thorough analysis of your skin, and then designs a program specifically for you. We are all completely unique genetic beings and our skin is no different. In addition, our skin is constantly changing as we age, thus changing its treatment requirements. A customized skin care program may include therapeutic office treatments such as micropeels, dermaplaning, and microdermabrasion in addition to daily product use including a cleanser, exfoliant, rejuvenating topical, and protection (sunblock.) The specific products used within this four-step treatment plan will vary depending on your age and skin type, but everyone benefits from all four steps.

The second set of treatment options in the bottom of the pyramid is the noninvasive lasers. This is a booming field of technological development with new lasers coming and going practically on a monthly basis. We could write an entire book on the various laser systems within this category but for the sake of this book, we will keep to those lasers we have found most useful in our practice. These include the Palomar ICON system, which offers an Intense Pulsed Light (or IPL) hand piece for removal of sunspots and redness (blood vessels), and the noninvasive fractional laser (Palomar 1540) for skin tightening, wrinkle reduction, and scar reduction. This system also has a hair removal application to remove unwanted hair on the face or body. The results we can accomplish with these technologies are very exciting. We do about 120 laser treatments per month (forty per week) in my office (including the IPL, the fractional, and laser hair removal) and we'll talk about them in chapter ten.

The third and last procedure in the noninvasive category is Ultherapy. This is an exciting new technology that employs focused ultrasound energy to tighten and lift the forehead, face, and neck. In fact, Ultherapy is the only FDA-approved technology for nonsurgical face lifting. We'll talk about Ultherapy in chapter eleven.

In the middle tier of the pyramid, we have our minimally invasive procedures—the injectables—which include Botulinum Toxin Type A (BOTOX®, Dysport® and XEOMIN™) and fillers. Don't let the word *toxin* frighten you. We'll discuss it fully in chapter eight. These procedures have become increasingly popular over the last decade. In our practice alone, we treat roughly one hundred patients per month with Botulinum Toxin Type A.

Colette, another patient for life, has had experience with all levels of the pyramid.

My Girlfriend Told Me I Needed Botox ... and That Was the Beginning

Colette

Age: 48

About twelve years ago, my husband and I went on vacation with another couple. I was on the beach with my girlfriend and happened to look up at the sun, and I was squinting. My girlfriend looked at me and said, "Oh my God. You need Botox." And that was the beginning. My friend led me by the hand and I did Botox.

When I met my husband he was in the fitness business, so we were really into being fit and eating well. These two things combined made me feel young. I'm plagued with Irish/Gaelic skin and it's not the best elasticity-wise. After two years of doing Botox I decided I wanted more. I felt younger on the inside than I looked on the outside and I wanted to tighten things up. Even though I was very fit, I felt like I had a bit of a double chin. I told my husband, "I just want to look like I did when you found me." We'd been together for ten years at that point.

Once I decided to have a face lift, I started asking my friends for referrals to plastic surgeons. We live in Toronto and there's one doctor who's the best of the best. They come from everywhere to see this guy, so I decided to go to him. It's my face and I wasn't about to look for the cheapest. I had seen someone whose face he'd done and she looked fabulous. I thought about it for only two months and then I had the surgery. (When I get something in my mind there's no stopping me.) After the surgery, the doctor said the result would be amazing. I also had a neck lift. I didn't do anything on my eyes or forehead...just the lower part of my face. I'm extremely happy with the result. On day three, my girlfriend wrapped my head in a scarf and made me go shopping with her. I was thinking, "Look at me. Look at me." I had very little bruising. I did have a numb face for a while—they told me this might happen—but it didn't matter because I was so happy.

A few years later, my husband and I started going to Florida in the winter. I thought it would be great to be able to get Botox—or anything else for that matter—while I was away. I started asking friends for referrals of doctors who do Botox in Southwest Florida. A friend of mine who spends winters in Florida overheard some women at the gym talking about Dr. Flaharty, so she asked them about him. They all raved about him, so my girlfriend and I both decided to try him. I've been seeing him for years now. I plan my Florida trips around my Botox. I get Botox when we first arrive in Florida and then I get it again right before we leave.

Since seeing Dr. Flaharty for Botox, I've also started doing more for my skin. I do photo rejuvenation. Being Irish, I had a lot of freckles and this laser treatment gets rid of the brown spots. I do my whole face twice a year. I get a monthly facial and dermaplaning. I also use Dr. Flaharty's Retin-A product. I do just a small amount of Restalyne to give me a little bit of a fuller lip. Dr. Flaharty is great at keeping you looking natural. I hate to brag, but I get told everywhere I go that I have beautiful skin. Even when I'm on vacation, if I go for a facial, the aesthetician tells me I have beautiful skin.

I agreed to do a television commercial for Dr. Flaharty. It was really fun because I was recognized everywhere I went. One day, in a grocery store, I heard someone whisper "I know her. She's an actress." I feel really great about my face. People freak out when I tell them how old I am. I'm so proud, I tell people before they have a chance to ask. I think about my mother at this age, or see pictures, and oh... what a difference. My kids' friends all say, "Your mom does not look her age."

My advice to others: it's okay to do these things. It will make you have more confidence, so why not? You must find a very good reputable doctor because there are a lot of flakes out there. You have to go for natural and not go over the top. The best way to find someone is through word of mouth. Personally, I want the whole package. I take great care of myself and I work hard at it. Initially, I wanted my face to match my body. Now, my face is my motivation to keep going to the gym.

We treat about the same number of patients with fillers as we do Botulinum Toxin Type A (the neurotoxins.) At Azul Cosmetic Surgery and Medical Spa, we offer three types of neurotoxins (Botox, Dysport and Xeomin) and several types of fillers. Both the neurotoxins and fillers are injected using fine-gauge needles. These procedures are done right in the office. It's not uncommon for a prospective patient to come into the office for a consultation, and decide on the spot to get neurotoxin injections, fillers, or both. Very often we're able to do the procedure right then and there. Many of our patients opt for the *Azul Liquid Face Lift*, a combination of Botulinum Toxin Type A and fillers, to give a fresh appearance to the face. The proper placement and amount of injectables is both a science and an art. You may have seen television personalities who've had a little too much Botulinum Toxin Type A injected, resulting in the "frozen face" appearance. Too much Botulinum Toxin Type A injected in the wrong place can result in a droopy brow or eyelid. You may have seen individuals with an unnatural, "Dr. Spock-like" lift of the eyebrows, the result of injections in the wrong place. In today's marketplace everybody and their brother is getting into injectables. Once again, you're advised to do your homework when choosing a practitioner. There is no substitute for experience. Recently a patient told me that while she was shopping at a boutique, the salesperson asked her about Botulinum Toxin Type A injections. When my patient inquired as to why the sales person had asked, the salesperson whispered, "We have someone doing injections in the back room today." Again, buyers beware.

Although the choices at the base and middle of the pyramid continue to evolve at a rapid pace, some results can be achieved only with surgery. At the apex of the pyramid, we have the surgical procedures: eyelid surgery, face and neck lift, endoscopic brow lift, fat transfer, chin augmentation, CO_2 laser skin resurfacing, and dermabrasion. As you will see in chapter eleven, the physical transformation achieved in just a few hours when performing a *panfacial* rejuvenation, which may include an endoscopic brow lift, eyelid surgery, a face and neck lift, fat transfer, and fillers—in a single procedure to rejuvenate the *entire* face at once—is a remarkable metamorphosis. I love the story of such a transformation from one of my patients, a highly successful salesperson. She'd been fired from her job by a new owner because she "looked too old." That's not supposed to happen in this day and age, but it does. After her face lift, she looked twenty years younger.   Subsequently, she re-entered the job market, was hired by a competitor, and became the top producing sales associate, earning twice what she made at her previous employer. "You go girl!"

By the way, a common misconception about the face lift is that it involves the entire face. It does not. A face lift involves only the lower portion of the face. Often we combine a face lift with a neck lift and brow lift, for a complete facial rejuvenation. In the last several years, there have been dramatic advances in the way face lifts are performed. A better understanding of facial anatomy in combination with endoscopic technology, utilizing smaller instruments and less invasive techniques, coupled with better anesthetic techniques, has led to quicker procedures, better results and less downtime. Another key advance in surgical rejuvenation comes with the awareness that much of facial aging is a result of volume loss (fat, muscle, and bone) resulting in facial deflation. In many cases to successfully rejuvenate the face we need to replace youthful volume with either fillers or fat transfer in addition to lifting and tightening. Combining these techniques gets us much closer to true three-dimensional rejuvenation of the face. Long gone are the days of the "pulled look." With proper advanced techniques complete and natural results can be achieved. In chapter twelve, we'll talk about the right time for surgery and take a closer look at the components of three-dimensional facial rejuvenation.

One thing to note: because technology is changing so fast, there's a fine line for doctors between jumping on the bandwagon, and ensuring a technology is solid before acquiring it. I like to keep up with the latest technology, but I don't always invest in it right away. I'm fortunate to have a personal network of like-minded doctors around the country. We share our knowledge and experience, which is invaluable when it comes to considering the addition of new technology to our menu of patient offerings.

My approach to facial rejuvenation is three-dimensional: it's about lifting, tightening and restoring volume. To achieve true three-dimensional rejuvenation of the face, we often combine several techniques. The specific techniques are individualized for each patient. Let's take a look at each of the procedures and treatments, one by one, beginning with skin care in the next chapter.

FIVE

· · · · · · · ·

Skin Care

Caring for the skin you're in

A
t the very bottom of our pyramid of facial rejuvenation is skin care. Taking good care of your skin will make a difference in how you look—to yourself and others. All other treatments and procedures, surgical and nonsurgical, will be enhanced by healthy, glowing skin. No matter your age, there are steps you can take to restore your skin's appearance and resilience: it's all about adopting a good daily regimen tailored to your skin, including protecting your skin from the sun. There's no need for your morning and evening routines to be complicated. In fact, in our practice, we believe in keeping skin care simple. Contrary to what some would believe, good skin care products do not have to cost a fortune.

WHAT IS SKIN CARE AND HOW DID IT BEGIN?

In a nutshell, skin care is ensuring that the largest organ of your body is well cared for. Of course, in this book we are talking specifically about the skin on your face. The history of skin care goes back to the Egyptians: it is reported that they made soap, soaked in milk baths, and moisturized with olive oil. In the Elizabethan era, those in the upper class sought to have pale skin, both to emulate the queen, and also to separate themselves from the working peasants who had darker skin, the result of working outdoors in the sun. To achieve this paleness, women used a lead-based whitening concoction. Not only did it make them pale, it made them sick. The use of lead-based beauty products continued into the second half of the 1800s when it was finally challenged in 1869 by the American Medical Association. In 1936, Ruth deForest Lamb, the chief education officer of the U.S. Food and Drug Administration wrote a book entitled *Chamber of Horrors.* In her book, Ms. Lamb disclosed stories of those who had suffered—and sometimes died—from the use of products containing unsafe ingredients. Her book revealed false advertising that promoted the use of such products, and included photographs of and letters written by the victims.[5] Two years later, in 1938, the Food, Drug and Cosmetics act was passed, putting cosmetics under the control of the FDA.

We've come a long way from the days of lead-based products. The first half of the 20th century witnessed a boom in the beauty industry, and along with it, the advent of companies such as Max Factor, Elizabeth Arden and L'Oreal. These companies introduced products such as face cream, makeup and mascara. Trends in beauty changed rapidly during the second half of the 1900s. Today, we recognize that skin care is at the foundation of beautiful, radiant skin.

SKIN CARE MYTHS AND MISCONCEPTIONS

In talking with hundreds of patients each month, we hear the same "skin care misconceptions" over and over:

- Skin care products are expensive.

- Complicated regimens with lots of products give the best results.

- If a product works for someone else, it will also work for you.

- All products with a certain ingredient are the same.

- The stronger the product, the better the result.

As you continue reading this chapter, I will dispel each of these myths.

THE FOUR STEPS OF SKIN CARE

When I started my practice, medical skin care in a physician's office was uncommon. As a result, many practices, including my own, didn't offer the cutting edge skin care products that have since become available to physicians. For the last ten years, we've offered the Azul Signature product line, our proprietary skin care line, and we're constantly committed to availing our clients to the very best, most sophisticated, state of the art skin care available today. Each product is made for us, to our specifications. We are dedicated to constant improvement in our skin care products to obtain the best results for our patients. Skin care is a great place to get started with facial rejuvenation for many of our patients because it's completely noninvasive. Getting medical-grade facials on a regular basis and using the right products for your skin will start to rebuild collagen and eliminate the dead cells on your skin's surface. It can make a dramatic improvement in both the quality and the appearance of your skin. If you choose to have other minimally invasive treatments or even surgery, proper skin care becomes an adjunct in terms of maintaining your investment. Skin care is a four-step process:

1. Cleanse

2. Exfoliate

3. Treat

4. Protect

Cleanse

The purpose of this first step in a skin care regimen is to remove makeup, sunscreen, dirt and oil. When it comes to cleansing, be sure to use a product that will cleanse without drying, as you can actually dehydrate your skin by utilizing the wrong cleanser. Regular bar soap is not meant for skin care. We offer four types of cleansers at Azul:

1. A sensitive skin cleanser is recommended for those with dry or sensitive skin

2. A gentle cleanser works on all skin types

3. An alpha-hydroxy cleanser helps cell turnover and is useful in an anti-aging regimen where a glycolic/lactic acid-based product is preferred for those with dry to normal skin

4. A glycolic acid/salicylic acid cleanser removes dead skin cells and is

preferred for those with acne or oily skin

Exfoliate

The exfoliation step helps to achieve healthy skin by removing the outer, damaged layer of skin, revealing the healthy skin below. It is this top layer of dead skin cells that causes the skin to look dull and dry. There are two types of exfoliants:

Mechanical exfoliants include the good old wash cloth, the newer sonic cleansing machines, and face scrubs.

Chemical exfoliants include enzyme-based products and peels.

Treat

The third step in your skin care regimen is to treat or nourish your skin. The key is to choose just the right active ingredient and concentration for your skin and your skin care goals. Here's a list of several of the active ingredients used in the Azul Signature product line:

- Vitamin C

- Vitamin E

- Green Tea

- Coenzyme Q-10

- Alpha Hydroxy Acids

- Vitamin A and Retinoids

- Hydroquinone

- Peptides

Each of the above ingredients serves a purpose. Not every ingredient is right for every individual.

Protect

The single most important thing you can do for your skin is to protect it. Sun exposure is the primary culprit when it comes to skin damage and skin cancer. UV radiation penetrates the skin, damaging skin cells. The result can be sunburn, discoloration, sun spots and dry skin. There are two types of sun protection products:

Physical blockers:
- Sunblock
- Hats
- Clothing
- Sun umbrellas

Chemical blockers:
- Sunscreen

SUNBLOCK VERSUS SUNSCREEN

Most people use the terms "sunblock" and "sunscreen" interchangeably. They aren't aware of the difference between the two: sunblock contains the *physical* ingredients zinc oxide and/or titanium dioxide. Sunblock does what it says: it *blocks* the sun's rays from reaching your skin, essentially acting as a wall between the sun and your skin. Sunscreen contains *chemical* ingredients that protect your skin by absorbing the ultraviolet light of the sun's rays. Sunscreens are not always well-tolerated by those with sensitive skin. I cannot stress sun protection enough: find a sunblock or sunscreen you like and wear it every day. It is also crucial to reapply your sunblock or sunscreen every two hours when in the sun. Whatever sunblock/sunscreen you use, it must block both UVA and UVB light. Sunblock containing zinc and titanium dioxide block both types of rays, but not all chemical sunscreens do. Be sure to look on the packaging for an indication that your sunscreen is "broad spectrum," which means it will block both UVA and UVB rays. In June 2012, the FDA passed new regulations allowing only those products that block both UVA and UVB to be labeled broad spectrum. The most exciting product we've developed over the last year is a fabulous sunblock that we call "Liquid Silk" because it truly glides onto your skin and feels wonderful. It's a physical blocker made of zinc and titanium dioxide; it's good for all types of skin, including sensitive skin, and blocks both UVA and UVB types of sunlight. The photo below may be a stretch, but I hope this visual leaves you with a vivid picture of the damage the sun can cause.

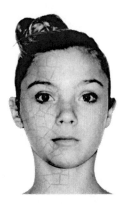

*This is Caroline. At her young age, she has the option of having
beautiful skin, or skin crackled by sun exposure.*

DEPARTMENT STORE, DRUG STORE, OR MEDICAL GRADE?

We all know skin care junkies who will try anything and everything and spend a small fortune doing so: they shop in drug stores, department stores, and on television. On the opposite side of the fence are the doubters who don't believe skin care products can make a difference. Then there are those in the middle: they're willing to try different products, but don't ask them to spend too much money. So what's the difference in skin care products you can purchase at a drug or department store, versus those you would purchase from a doctor's office?

The difference between products you can purchase "over the counter" at a drug store or department store, and medical-grade skin care products is the concentration of ingredients. Medical-grade products—which can be purchased only through a physician's office—contain a higher concentration of the ingredients that will make the most difference to your skin. **It's all about pure ingredients and scientific delivery systems.** Ordinary products penetrate only the top layer of skin, and contain fewer of the ingredients that sustain cellular health. Medical-grade products are stronger and penetrate deeper into the middle layer of the skin, where collagen and elastin are present and where new skin cells are produced. **Medical-grade products deliver maximum concentrations of the healing ingredients known to promote skin health: they improve your skin from the inside out.**

This is not to say that over the counter products are bad; they're just not as effective. For example, one of the complaints my medical aestheticians hear most often is, "My skin looks dull." Generally, this is because of dead skin cells on the surface of the skin. Retinoid creams help to remove that layer of dead skin cells, and to build new collagen beneath. (The secret to keeping a glow to your skin as you age is to use products that will remove that layer of dead skin cells on the surface.) When you use medical-grade, or prescription retinoid products such as Tretinoin (Retin-A,) you will begin to see the effect in as little as two months. An over the counter option may take twice as long and the result will not be as dramatic, or...you may not see a change at all.

WHAT'S THE COST OF SKIN CARE?

When it comes to skin care products, more is not better. Some of our products are priced as low as $20. Our average patient spends $100–$200 for a full regimen of skin care products that will last around four months. It seems like a bargain compared to the extravagantly-packaged, over-priced lotions and potions you might purchase in a department store. Please visit our online store to see our skin care line: http://store.azulbeauty.com/

WHAT ABOUT MAKEUP?

We offer the Jane Iredale mineral-based product line and recommend it to our post-surgery patients. It's crucial that only hypo-allergenic products be used on post-surgery skin. This particular company got its start as a pure mineral makeup product to cover redness and bruising after surgery. Not only do our post-surgery patients use this makeup, but many of our skin care patients use it as well.

WHAT DOES A MEDICAL AESTHETICIAN DO?

Most of our patients are introduced to our medical aesthetician when they make an appointment for a facial or as part of a skin care evaluation. The first thing our aesthetician will do is take a detailed history—including any previous treatments and procedures—and perform a thorough evaluation of your skin's condition. She will also review any skin care products you are presently using. Depending on your goals for your skin and the condition of your skin, she will then recommend a course of action including at-home skin care and in-office treatments. Of course, the choice is yours as to what you will do.

Our aesthetician-administered in-office treatments include medical-grade facials, dermaplaning and microdermabrasion, as well as glycolic, salicylic and TCA peels. The cost of these treatments with our medical aesthetician ranges from $95–$150. Our medical aesthetician is also certified in the application of permanent makeup for permanent brow liner and eyeliner.

Medical-Grade Facial

The facials we provide in our office—while relaxing—are less about pampering than they are about providing a medical-grade, transformative treatment for your skin. Our signature facial is a therapeutic deep-cleansing facial, customized for you. Specific nutrients and ingredients treat your skin at its deepest level without being too aggressive.

Dermaplaning Facial

Dermaplaning is a light exfoliation of the facial skin with a blade. Your face is cleansed before the dermaplaning. Moisturizer and sunscreen are applied after the treatment. The dermaplaning facial takes about thirty minutes and there is no downtime. After the treatment, your skin is very smooth, providing for a flawless makeup application. Dermaplaning is a wonderful monthly maintenance treatment.

Microdermabrasion Facial

An exfoliating process, microdermabrasion has been around for a long time. Best for thicker or oily skin, microdermabrasion essentially polishes the outer layer of the skin. Dermplaning is included in the microdermabrasion treatment, as is extraction, massage and a mask. Microdermabrasion is a great monthly maintenance treatment.

Micropeel

A micropeel is a light chemical peel performed with an acid, typically glycolic acid or salicylic acid. (Our medical aesthetician chooses the acid appropriate for your skin.) Your face is cleansed and dermaplaned in preparation for the peel. This treatment also includes extractions, steam, a facial massage, mask and moisturizer. There is no downtime with a micropeel, and no post-treatment peeling. It takes about an hour. You will leave our office with glowing skin.

Medical Peel

Medical (chemical) peels increase cellular turnover, refining the epidermis. Medical peels treat varying skin conditions including sun damage, acne, and sensitive, dry or oily skin. You may have heard these peels called by different names: TCA or Jessner, for example. The treatment takes half an hour and the type of peel selected is based on your specific skin condition. You will have mild flaking for 5–7 days following your medical peel, after which your skin will be renewed and refreshed. It is suggested that you have a facial one month after your peel.

The TCA Under-Eye Peel

Tricholoracetic acid, or TCA for short, can be used for both light and medium peels, depending upon the strength of acid used. The TCA under-eye peel, administered by a doctor, is effective at eliminating crepey skin and fine lines under the eyes. A cotton swab is used to apply three to five coats of the TCA solution to the under-eye area. There is mild stinging, which resolves quickly with cool compresses. The skin appears frosty immediately after the solution is applied. The area is then covered with Vaseline.

There is downtime associated with the TCA peel as the skin under your eyes turns reddish brown and then peels over the course of a week. During that time you must avoid the sun and keep the area covered with Vaseline until it is completely healed.

THE BOTTOM LINE

Good skin care truly makes a difference. If you intend to have other facial rejuvenation treatments, the result will be better when the quality and appearance of your skin is improved with good skin care. Many of our patients have breathed sighs of relief when they've learned the difference good skin care can make, and how reasonably-priced it is. One patient, who admits to being a former skin care-product junkie, estimates that she has saved about $500 per year since she began using our skin care products. Not only has she saved money, but she saves time as well: she's no longer drawn to the shopping channels on television, or the counters in department stores. And... she claims her skin looks better than ever before. I think a good way to end this chapter on skin care is with a story from one of our patients...

My Skin Cancer Resulted in the Opening of a Door to a Whole New Universe

Ellie

Age: 50

Last year, I discovered a "spot" under my right eye. I assumed it was nothing serious, but decided to visit my dermatologist to have it checked out. A biopsy revealed the spot to be a basal-cell carcinoma[6], a form of skin cancer. My dermatologist informed me that the basal cell would have to be surgically removed and that he could perform the surgery. (My dermatologist is also a Mohs[7] surgeon.)

The surgery to remove the basal-cell left a significant hole in my face. My dermatologist referred me to Dr. Flaharty to do the "clean up and correction" after the Mohs surgery. From my first visit with Dr. Flaharty, I felt very well held. My face and how I look is important, as it is for everyone. Dr. Flaharty did the correction: I ended up with stitches from the outside corner of my eye, to the inside corner of my eye where it meets my nose, and all the way down the side of my nose. I was not pretty to look at, though I have to say the cut and stitches were perfect, and matched with my natural facial contours.

Post-surgery, I went to Dr. Flaharty for quite a while. He paid a lot of careful attention to how my face was healing and how I was feeling about it. There was a lot of red and raised-up scarring along the side of my nose. Dr. Flaharty recommended some laser treatments—performed by his physician assistant—to help reduce the redness and swelling. Dr. Flaharty is a perfectionist in the good sense of the word. Even after the laser treatments, he wasn't satisfied with the way my face looked. (I actually thought it was okay.) I had another set of laser treatments to facilitate the growth of more collagen.

Even after the second set of laser treatments, Dr. Flaharty wanted to make the scar a little more even where it was showing, so he used a bit of Restylane. He is an amazing physician. His talent impresses me, but it's really Dr. Flaharty's manner, his deep care, and his sensitivity to his patients that truly amaze me. If Dr. Flaharty hadn't fixed my face after the Mohs surgery, I would have looked like Frankenstein. I'm so grateful I don't have a big scar. I'm absolutely delighted and I don't know what I would have done without him. I recommend him all the time.

During the time I had the stitches—about three weeks—I wasn't able to clean my face the way I normally would. I had massive stitches. The area was swollen and tender, and I didn't want to mess things up. During one visit to Dr. Flaharty's office, his nurse suggested I might want to get a facial and Dr. Flaharty agreed. I'd had one or two facials before, but they were the pampering-type of facials. I didn't understand the benefits of what a good facial can do for you. I decided to give it a try. Dr. Flaharty's medical aesthetician is excellent and loves her work. Since this was all new to me, she was gentle and sensitive to my needs, but it wasn't just a relaxing facial: the pores in my nose were all plugged up around where the stitches had been. The cleaning of my pores was a little painful during that first facial because I had so much build-up in my face.

After the first facial, I bought a package and started getting facials every three to four weeks. I continue to get facials on a regular basis. I love having them and I feel so much better. Now when I go, there's so much less of the work of cleaning out pores. Today, my skin looks so different: healthier, better color, and no clogged pores anymore. I used to love being out in the sun and having the sun on my face, not just for the tan, but for the way it feels to have the sun on my face. I felt if I didn't have a suntan, I looked washed out. Today my skin is so much more healthy-looking: it's clear and has a natural glow without putting on any makeup. I must admit I'm not a makeup person. I wear mascara and that's it.

A couple of months after the surgery, I saw my sister-in-law. She took one look at me and knew something was different. She actually asked if I'd had a face lift. It all started because of the surgery, and now I will take good care of my skin and get facials for the rest of my life.

I've received an education and now understand the different types of skin care products. I use a special cleanser for my type of skin and a sonic facial brush I purchased from Dr. Flaharty's office. I use their treatment pads for exfoliating and I really love their sunscreen: it's so silky.

I never would have thought of this before, but now I'm sort of thinking I might move into other things. Now I notice more: the creases between my eyebrows. I'm not going to do anything today or tomorrow, but my awareness has been raised. I've learned about permanent makeup, and laser treatments for brown spots, blood vessels, and redness. Then of course there's Botox and fillers. It's a completely different universe for me.

My advice to others is to take care of your skin. Go to a medical aesthetician and go with quality products, because that's what works. A lot of people see things on TV or they try different products from drugstores or the shopping channels. If you go with a place like Azul— where the people really know what they're doing—you'll get real results. They don't push you into products you don't want.

I've become an advocate for skin care and I want to spread the word. People find out because of others' good experiences. I never thought about facials or skin care. I never knew anything about it. The assumption people make is that skin care is only for those who have a lot of money. That's not true. Skin care is for everyone, not just the rich and famous. That's why I'm so passionate about it. One last thing: facials are not about pampering... they're about skin care, with care being the underlined word.

SIX

······

BOTULINUM TOXIN TYPE A

Five-minute magic

With over four million injections, treatment with Botulinum Toxin Type A (the neurotoxins) was the number one nonsurgical cosmetic procedure in 2011. "Botox" has become a household word. While a majority of people have heard the word, "Botox," I suspect most people don't really know much about it other than the fact that it's used to smooth out forehead wrinkles and frown lines, and...that it's a *toxin.* While the word *toxin* sounds scary, the injection of Botulinum Type A is one of the safest cosmetic procedures: it has a history of more than 100 years and today is considered the gold standard for softening frown lines, forehead wrinkles, and crow's feet. It can be used alone, or in combination with fillers or even surgery.

WHAT EXACTLY IS BOTULINUM TOXIN TYPE A AND HOW LONG HAS IT BEEN AROUND?

Botulinum Toxin Type A is a neurotoxin, a purified protein derived from *Clostridium botulinum,* which is a type of bacterium. While I wouldn't normally bore you with a history lesson, I think the history of Botulinum Toxin Type A is important to the understanding of its safety, which goes back to 1895, when the bacterium was identified. Researchers have been fascinated by the potential of this bacterium ever since. In the 1950s, it was discovered that Botulinum Toxin Type A can reduce muscle spasms. Over the next forty years, researchers continued to study this neurotoxin, discovering a number of medical uses. In 1989, Allergan Pharmaceuticals introduced Botox as the first botulinum toxin approved by the Food and Drug Administration (FDA) to treat crossed eyes and eyelid spasms. In 2000, Botox was approved by the FDA to treat muscle spasms in the neck, resulting from a condition called cervical dystonia. In 2002, the FDA approved BOTOX˚ Cosmetic (the same formulation as Botox) for frown lines between the eyebrows. Botox celebrated twenty years of FDA approval in 2010. Research on Botox continues and the indications for its use continue to expand. In addition to its cosmetic use, Botulinum Toxin Type A is used today to treat muscle stiffness, reduce chronic migraines and certain types of glandular activity such as excessive sweating.

Botulinum Toxin Type A (BOTOX˚Cosmetic, Dysport˚ and XEOMIN™) is the most popular family of injectable cosmetic products available. It comes in a sterile vial as a freeze-dried powder. A prescribed amount of saline is injected into the vial to make a solution ready for use. The resultant liquid contains tiny amounts of the highly purified botulinum toxin protein refined from the bacterium. The product is administered in small injections to temporarily weaken the muscle by blocking the electrical signals between the nerve and muscle.

THE MOST POPULAR COSMETIC NONSURGICAL PROCEDURE

Since 2000, Botulinum Toxin Type A has been the most popular cosmetic nonsurgical procedure. In 2011, it was the top nonsurgical cosmetic procedure in the U.S. among both women and men, with 2,619,739 injections (BOTOX˚Cosmetic and Dysport˚ combined,) performed by physicians and 4,030,318 performed by physicians, physician assistants and nurses. Men received 10.1 percent of those injections.[8]

HOW MANY COMPANIES MANUFACTURE THE NEUROTOXINS?

Botox by Allergan was the original product, approved for cosmetic use in 2002. Dysport, distributed by Medicis, is the leading competitor to Allergan's Botox, and was FDA approved in 2009. Dysport's biggest claim is that it starts working sooner and lasts longer than other neurotoxins.

Xeomin, manufactured by Merz Pharmaceuticals, is the newest addition to the Botulinum Toxin Type A family. Originally used to treat neck and eyelid spasms, Xeomin has recently been introduced in the cosmetic world after being approved by the FDA in July of 2011.

WHAT CONCERNS CAN BOTULINUM TOXIN TYPE A INJECTIONS TREAT?

- frown lines between the eyebrows

- forehead wrinkles

- crow's feet

- frown lines at the corners of the mouth

- upper lip lines

- neck bands

- chin dimpling

In chapter one, we talked about the two different types of wrinkles: dynamic and static. Dynamic wrinkles result from muscle action. There are many facial muscles responsible for expression and facial animation. These muscles are important for nonverbal communication, but they can cause unwanted lines and creases such as frown lines, forehead creases, crow's feet, lip lines, and neck bands. Using the neurotoxins, we selectively weaken certain muscles that are used for facial expression, thereby smoothing the overlying skin and resulting in a more youthful, refreshed appearance.

Botulinum Toxin Type A is injected in tiny amounts using a narrow-gauge needle directly into the overactive muscle. The neurotoxin diffuses into the muscle, temporarily weakening it. There is a great deal of sophistication that can be applied to these injections: the key to success is knowing exactly where and how much to inject. Cosmetic surgeons are extremely well versed in facial anatomy. Understanding this anatomy is paramount in being able to administer the neurotoxins for the right facial expressions. For example, there are differences in the facial structures of men and women, and a practitioner must have a solid understanding of such nuances in order to achieve a flawless result. In addition, men and women often have different cosmetic goals. (See chapter twelve, *For Men Only.*) The injection of Botulinum Toxin Type A should take these differences into account. Our patient, David, gets Botox for forehead wrinkles and crow's feet.

I Wondered Why My Friend Didn't Have Crow's Feet Like Me

David

Age: 35

A couple of years ago, I noticed that a friend of mine—who is exactly the same age as I am—looked really terrific. I wondered why she didn't have crow's feet and forehead lines like me. I asked what she was doing to look so young and she replied, "Botox!" I was really curious to try it, but hesitant at the same time. Being in the beauty industry, a daily topic of discussion with my clients and the other stylists is how to look one's best, so I started asking everyone about Botox. I discovered I wasn't the only one who was afraid to take the plunge. It was fear of the unknown more than anything, though I was also concerned about whether it would hurt. I finally decided to just do it. I loved the result and I also loved that everyone noticed how much younger I looked. I now get Botox on a regular basis. I can tell when it starts to wear off, and I make my appointment right away.

My advice to anyone considering Botox is to call Dr. Flaharty's office— or, if you're not here in Southwest Florida, to find a great doctor—and take the plunge. Don't put it off. I would have done it sooner if I'd known how good the results would be. I also think maintenance is easier if you keep up on the schedule, and you actually need less Botox.

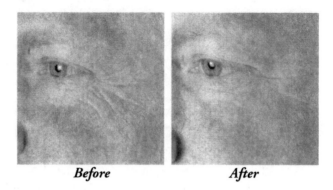

Before   *After*

**These photos show typical crow's feet around the eyes before and after
neurotoxin injections. The patient is not squinting in either photo.**

IS ANY PREPARATION REQUIRED BEFORE GETTING NEUROTOXIN INJECTIONS?

No, you do not have to prepare in any way before getting these injections. In fact, patients will often come in for a consult and end up getting their injections at the same time. This is a true lunch-time procedure.

How Is The Treatment Done?

Botox, Dysport and Xeomin injections are typically performed in the office setting. They are administered with a series of injections in the area to be treated, using the narrowest gauge needle available.

How Long Does It Take?

If numbing cream is used, your appointment will be about thirty minutes. If numbing cream is not used, the appointment will be around fifteen minutes.

What Is The Pain Factor?

Typically the treatment areas are numbed with a topical anesthetic cream for fifteen to twenty minutes. Some patients decline the numbing cream. Even though we use a very tiny needle, there is some stinging and burning with the injections and the numbing cream reduces that discomfort. The injections are very quick and it takes only a few minutes to treat the entire face. There is minimal discomfort after the procedure.

What Are The Side Effects?

All medicines may cause side effects. Most people have no problems with the neurotoxins, though side effects can occur. The most common side effect is bruising, redness and pain at the injection site. Sometimes patients complain of a headache or tingly feeling immediately after Botox injections. Optimal cosmetic improvement is achieved by placing the right amount of Botox in the right location. Undesirable outcomes such as the "frozen face" from too much Botox, droopy eyelids, and unnaturally shaped or droopy eyebrows can occur with inappropriate placement of the product. All neurotoxin side effects are temporary.

Is There Any Downtime?

There is no downtime after receiving Botulinum Toxin Type A injections. You can leave our office and go straight to lunch, dinner, or back to work.

How Long Will It Last?

The neurotoxins do not work immediately; typically the full effect can be seen 7–14 days after treatment. On average, Botulinum Toxin Type A lasts 3–4 months. Some patients find their result lasting as long as six months. Most of my neurotoxin patients come for treatments two times per year. You can expect to need more treatments the first year, sometimes three or four. Many of my patients find they need less Botulinum Toxin Type A as time goes on, because the muscles become less active.

In the hands of a skilled, experienced practitioner, Botulinum Toxin Type A can make a striking difference in a patient's overall appearance. Combined with medical-grade skin care and additional interventions like fillers, Botox repeatedly earns high marks and is among the "gold standards" in achieving a refreshed, natural, youthful look and feel for countless men and women. Let's take a look at some of the other technologies that have their own rightful place in that proverbial fountain of youth.

SEVEN

· · · · · · · · · · · · · · ·

FILLERS

The new all-stars

Facial fillers are a powerful weapon in our fight against facial aging. It is now well recognized that much of facial aging is the result of fat and soft tissue loss, which causes a hollowed or deflated look to the face. When I conduct seminars at my office, I enjoy showing a photo of my three daughters when they were five, eight and ten years old. I tell my audience to notice the round cheeks and full lips of youth. Once upon a time, it was thought that lines, wrinkles, and laxity were the culprits that make us look older.In the world of cosmetic facial rejuvenation, we've come to realize it's not only the lines and wrinkles that age us: it's the hollowing, flatness, and thinning of our face through global fat loss. Fillers do exactly what they say: they *fill* facial lines, wrinkles and hollows, as well as re-volumize the face. There are a number of different fillers available on the market today and the list is growing almost daily. The most frequently used fillers contain all-natural substances including hyaluronic acid and calcium phosphate, both of which are found naturally in our bodies. We use a number of different fillers in our practice, with most of them containing these all-natural substances.

WHAT CONCERNS CAN FILLERS TREAT?

Since much of facial aging is the result of global volume loss, facial fillers are now being used everywhere on the face to restore youthful contouring and volume. Specific problem areas include:

- Hollowing and/or dark circles under the eyes

- Frown lines

- Nasolabial folds

- Marionette lines

- Wrinkling or folds

- Thin lips

- Sunken cheekbones

- Hollow temples

- Deflated eyebrows

- Weakened jawline

- Overall facial deflation

WHAT ARE THE DIFFERENT TYPES OF FILLERS?

There are two classes of fillers: volume replacement fillers (Hyaluronic Acid fillers) and stimulatory fillers. The volume replacement fillers create volume as they settle into the tissues. Gradually—over the course of months or years—these fillers dissolve and that volume is lost once again. The stimulatory fillers compel the body to create new collagen. Volume is created through the combination of the filler material and the new collagen that is built around it. Stimulatory fillers can last for a number of years. Let's take a look at both types of fillers in more detail.

Volume Replacement Fillers: Restylane®, Perlane®, JUVÉDERM®, BELOTERO®

The volume replacement fillers are all made from hyaluronic acid, or HA, for short. These are the most commonly used fillers, both in the United States and worldwide. In 2011, HA fillers were the second most popular cosmetic nonsurgical procedure, with over 1.5 million injections performed in the U.S.[9] Restylane was the first stabilized HA filler on the market. Since that time, a number of additional HA fillers have been approved by the FDA including Perlane, Juvederm, Belotero and others. This list continues to grow as companies pursue new forms of HA to address the various facial aging needs.

Why Are HAs So Important?

HA fillers are presently the most important class of fillers. I call them the work-horse fillers. Hyaluronic acid, a lubricating protein that attracts and retains water, is a protein that's naturally present in our skin and joints. Hyaluronic acid is made synthetically in a laboratory. It's sterile and identical to our native proteins, so there is no risk of being allergic to these products. HAs are clear and gel-like, and can be injected at any level of the face from the skin down to the bone and everywhere in between, making them very versatile fillers. HA fillers are soft and pliable and can be molded into the desired shape or contour once placed in the face. HA fillers are the only class of fillers that are reversible. (In the rare case where eliminating the HA filler would be necessary, an enzyme called hyaluronidase is injected to dissolve the hyaluronic acid filler.) This degree of control and reversibility makes HA fillers very attractive to both patients and physicians.

In my practice, HAs are used for mild to moderate facial lines, folds, and wrinkles and less often for deeper lifting, volumizing, and contouring. Because they are clear, malleable, and reversible, HA fillers are also used for delicate areas including the lower eyelids, lips, and fine lines. As the most versatile filler, HAs can be used anywhere including nasolabial folds, marionette lines, temples, cheeks, lower face, jawline, lip lines, frown lines between the brows and facial scars. HA fillers are often used in conjunction with the neurotoxins (Botox, Dysport or Xeomin) to address dynamic wrinkles and lines, folds, and hollows all in a single treatment. When rejuvenating the face with a combination of fillers and neurotoxins, we call it a *Liquid Face Lift*. We'll discuss the *Azul Liquid Face Lift* in the next chapter.

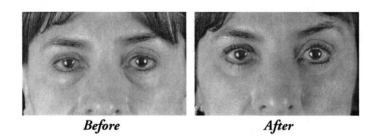

Before   *After*

***The hollowness and dark circles under the eyes
are gone after the use of HA fillers.***

The Future of HA Fillers

The genesis of HA fillers arms the physician with different formulations to address different needs. For example, a thinner HA may be appropriate for the fine lines of the upper lip while a heavier, thicker HA may be better to restore volume to the cheeks, temples, or jawline. One thing is certain, we will see new forms of HA arriving on the scene in the months and years to come.

Stimulatory Fillers: RADIESSE®, Artefill©, Sculptra®

The second class of fillers are the stimulatory fillers. Radiesse is one such filler: it has calcium phosphate microspheres suspended in a water based gel. Radiesse is considered natural because calcium phosphate occurs naturally in our bodies. When injected, the gel disappears in approximately two months, but the calcium phosphate beads remain, and the body grows collagen around the beads. The complex of beads and collagen will last several years. Radiesse is placed deeper into the face than the hyaluronic acid fillers. The primary use of Radiesse is to smooth deeper nasolabial folds and marionette lines, and to add volume to the cheeks and jawline. Radiesse is often used in combination with an HA filler for optimal results that last 6 months to 2 years, depending on the volume and location.

Artefill is similar to Radiesse in that it is a stimulatory filler, but unlike the other fillers, it's not natural. Artefill is composed of poly methyl methacrylate (PMMA) beads suspended in a purified bovine (cow) collagen gel. The inert beads of PMMA are well-tolerated in the body, but are permanent as the body cannot break down or dissolve this material. The bovine collagen is cow collagen which is not identical to human collagen. Approximately three percent of the population may react to bovine collagen; therefore, we need to do a skin test before injecting Artefill so we can ensure there is no reaction to it. If a patient reacts to the skin test, we will not use this product. The benefit of Artefill is that your body will never break down the PMMA beads. The minute beads are the size of a red blood cell, so you don't see them or feel them at all. When injected into the tissues, new collagen will grow and envelope the PMMA beads. The complex of beads and collagen will last for years. It provides both immediate and long-lasting results by visibly correcting the wrinkles, and providing structural support for the skin. Artefill is the first and only permanent, injectable filler which is FDA-approved for the treatment of nasolabial folds (smile lines.)

Sculptra® (poly-L-Lactic acid) is a third type of stimulatory filler. This product is not routinely found in the body. Sculptra is usually injected in a series of three treatments over several months. The material will stimulate a reaction in your tissues leading to the formation of collagen, thus adding volume to the face. Sculptra is primarily used for creating global volume in the cheek and temple areas. The results last several years.

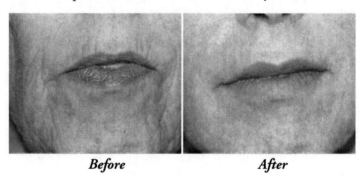

Before   **After**

*In this patient, a combination of Radiesse and Restylane was used
to rejuvenate the creases and folds around the mouth area.*

An Important Note

The face is a dynamic, evolving structure that is changing every day. Patients often inquire about "something more permanent" when discussing treatment options. The reality is that nothing we do to the face will stop these ongoing changes. For example, the PMMA beads of Artefill will indeed be permanent, but all the surrounding tissue will continue to evolve and change and as such, some of the effects of Artefill will be lost over time. (This is no different than what happens with a face lift.)

Is Any Preparation Required?

Avoiding aspirin or other blood thinners can reduce your risk of bruising after fillers. We recommend patients clear their schedules so they can use ice intermittently for a few hours after receiving the filler injections.

How Is It Done?

The injection of fillers is an in-office procedure. After cleansing your face, we apply a numbing cream and allow that to work for 15–20 minutes. The numbing cream is then removed with an anti-bacterial cleanser and the fillers are injected into the area to be treated using a fine-gauge needle. Ice is used intermittently to reduce discomfort. I like to inject a small amount, pause to look at the result, and then inject a little more. I do one side of the face first, and then I do the other side to match. Sometimes the amount of filler required on one side of the face is different than on the other side. This is the beauty of fillers: we can place volume where we want it. Injecting fillers is a very gratifying and artistic experience for me: I am able to create volume and three-dimensionally revitalize the face with immediate results. Patients also see the result right away. In fact, I often have a patient look in a mirror after one side of the face is done so they can see the improvement.

How Long Does It Take?

The average filler appointment is about sixty minutes, allowing time for the numbing cream to work, and for the injections.

What's The Pain Factor?

Filler injections generally cause minimal discomfort. A numbing cream is applied before the injections and ice is applied during and immediately after the injections to minimize any pain, swelling, and potential bruising.

What Are The Side Effects?

Side effects of fillers are generally mild and temporary. Redness, swelling, and bruising are the most common and typically resolve in a few days to a week. Makeup can be used immediately after fillers. Palpable or visible lumps and bumps can occur, but these are generally avoidable with good technique and are temporary. More serious complications of infection or vascular occlusion have been reported but are exceedingly rare and generally involve fillers that are not comprised of substances found naturally in the body.

Is There Any Downtime?

There is no downtime with fillers. If you happen to have any redness, swelling, or bruising, you can use makeup immediately after the treatment. Most patients return to normal activities right away. The more filler you have placed, the more likely you are to have some visible signs of the procedure. Many patients request fillers prior to a big event. We recommend getting your fillers a minimum of two weeks, and preferably one month prior to the event. We certainly do not recommend fillers right before a big social event. Your best results will be visible at one month, once the fillers have settled into place and any swelling has completely resolved.

How Long Does It Last?

The results of fillers are immediate and can last six months to several years depending on the treatment area and type of filler used. In high-movement areas such as around the mouth, fillers are broken down more quickly and often disappear over six months to one year. Artefill is an exception as the beads cannot be broken down, so the result is longer-lasting. In low-movement areas such as under the eyes or the cheeks, fillers often last for years and can even be permanent. Some of my patients have reported that they remain pleased with their under-eyes ten years after having had HA fillers injected.

We've taken a look at the benefits of fillers and we've talked about the neurotoxins: Botox, Dysport and Xeomin. While Botox has been around for quite a while, facial fillers have become more popular in the last ten years since new fillers have entered the marketplace. Years ago, the only filler we had was bovine collagen. It was thin, watery and only lasted a few weeks. The newer fillers are thicker and longer-lasting, opening up exciting possibilities. In the next chapter, we'll go a little deeper (so to speak!) and explore the synergistic power of using neurotoxins and fillers in a single treatment in what we call the Azul Liquid Face Lift.

EIGHT

· · · · · · · · · · ·

THE LIQUID FACE LIFT

Restoring volume for a more youthful you

Something that has become very popular at Azul Cosmetic Surgery and Medical Spa is the Azul Liquid Face Lift, which combines neurotoxins with fillers to rejuvenate the face.

In chapter one, I talked about aging. We used to think aging was all about wrinkles and laxity and thus, a face lift was all about tightening and lifting. We've come to realize more recently that aging is not only about wrinkles and laxity, but it's also very much about loss of volume in the face. (I think by now you're getting this message!) As we age, we get more hollow and sunken. When we add volume back into the face with fillers, it can have an amazing result. We want a more youthful appearance, but it should be soft, because youthful beauty is soft. It's not tight and it certainly isn't flat, hollow, or deflated.

The Liquid Face Lift offers wonderful possibilities with the combination of neurotoxins to relax the muscles and fillers to restore volume. Different techniques are used depending on the concerns of the patient. One of the most frequently requested areas patients want smoothed out is the vertical lines between the eyebrows. A couple of tiny injections of Botox diffused into the muscle relaxes it, and not only smooths out the frown lines, but actually lifts up the brow and smooths the skin as well. A different technique with neurotoxins will result in a nice lifting of the lateral brow. The combination of lifting the brow and smoothing those frown lines is something that's very popular with men and women. Another benefit of Botox is that it shrinks down some of the sebaceous glands which further smooths the skin's surface.

Technique is critical when it comes to injecting neurotoxins. For example, too much in the wrong place can result in a droopy brow as opposed to a raised brow. It's also important to note the differences in men versus women: men's eyebrows go straight across. Women's eyebrows are arched. Turn up your antennae and start looking at faces all around you: your friends and neighbors, television personalities, people on the street. I've noticed some male television personalities in particular, who've had a little too much Botox injected in the wrong places. Both science and art are involved in the Liquid Face Lift. Knowledge of facial anatomy is essential to injecting the right quantities of Botox and fillers, and injecting them in the right places.

Once the frown lines, forehead lines and crow's feet have been smoothed out with neurotoxins, the next step in the Liquid Face lift is to fill deeper folds and add volume back into the face using fillers. Areas in which fillers are used to add volume include the lips, cheeks, temples, jawline, frown lines, folds and creases around the mouth, and dark circles under the eyes. Since loss of volume from the face is global, we're finding that adding fillers anywhere on the face can help turn back the hands of time.

A pleasing and natural facial rejuvenation is very often dependent upon a practitioner's expert knowledge in combining therapies to achieve a natural, flawless result. As in everything in life, there is no substitute for experience.

One of the stories I love to tell is that of a former nun in her early eighties. I had done eyelid surgery for her years earlier. She came back to see me and told me that in two weeks she was getting married to a younger man. Her fiancé told her she "didn't need anything," but she wanted to look her very best on her wedding day. We came up with a great plan using a combination of Botox and fillers. She was thrilled with the results and all of us in the office made her promise to stop in and show us wedding photos, which she did after their honeymoon. There was a little lesson for me in this experience: the desire to look and feel good knows no age, and it shouldn't.

The Liquid Face Lift makes a real difference for our patients, just like it did for Jenna.

I Looked Tired and Serious All the Time

Jenna

Age: 52

Coming up on my 49th birthday, I was face to face with a mid-life crisis. I was newly divorced and miserable and a sibling had been diagnosed with terminal cancer. I had two thoughts, "How did I get to this place?" and "Life is too precious and short to waste any more time on things that are not important." As a career woman, I had thrown everything into my work and ignored my own happiness and that of my family. I had been in search of "being successful in the corporate world someday" at the expense of "being happy today." I was not happy, yet I didn't even recognize it because my own needs had been buried so deeply, while chasing an empty dream. So at that point, I decided to adopt the method they recommend by the airlines: "put on your oxygen mask first before helping others." If I was in a better place, then my capacity to help others and open my heart would also be greater.

Always attractive and naturally slim, I had progressively put on weight and was not exercising or eating particularly well. As I looked in the mirror, I saw someone I did not even recognize, physically, emotionally or spiritually. I knew I needed to do something about it; how I would come out of this crisis was totally and 100 percent up to me.

I knew the easiest thing to start with was my appearance, and I knew it would help me feel better about myself. I started exercising and eating right and within a month I had gotten in really good shape and dropped almost twenty pounds. The exercise alone helped my mental state, and being able to wear clothes that looked good on me was also rewarding. Simultaneously, I started working fewer hours and really made an effort to connect with my family and friends, all while going to church or meditating every morning to replenish my spirit.

With my body in shape and my spirit beginning to come alive again, I needed to address my face: I looked tired or serious all the time because of my frown lines and my face had become hollow with the weight loss. I'd had Botox before and liked the result, but I had not kept up with it, nor had I ever tried any other cosmetic treatments. One of my friends told me she had recently had something called a *Liquid Face Lift* with Dr. Flaharty, and she was absolutely thrilled with the result. I decided to make an appointment and see if I could make my face match my now more-youthful body.

I asked Dr. Flaharty about the Liquid Face Lift. He agreed that it was a good option for me. The nurses applied numbing cream, and I waited about thirty minutes. From the time they came in the room with the injections, the whole procedure took only about ten minutes. The most painful part was the Botox, but it was hardly anything worse than a bee sting. Fillers under the eyes and in the cheek area are easy. In fact you can't feel anything after the numbing cream. I had some minor bruising afterwards, but was able to hide it with makeup.

The result was dramatic, and I was thrilled. In fact, I was at a party shortly afterwards and went up to a couple that I had met a few months earlier and reintroduced myself. They looked at me and after a few seconds of silence, the wife said "Oh my gosh, you don't even look like the same person!" I replied, "Well, I've been working out." I didn't share that I really was a different person.

Today, I am no longer the robotic box-checker married to my job. Yes, I have responsibilities like everyone, but I try to put aside time every day to take care of myself, and to tell my family that I love them. I find joy in living in the moment, including watching my beloved cat be a complete goofball. The physical transformation that I was able to make helped me bring other parts of my life into balance. I will continue to have procedures to enhance my looks, as it has made a difference in my happiness and self-confidence. In fact, I think I'll have Dr. Flaharty do my eyelids soon. For anyone considering getting a procedure done I say, "Do it, do it, do it!" Find the right doctor, certainly, and do the procedure that is right for you, but don't be afraid. The benefits far outweigh the risks.

Everything we've discussed has its place in your personal quest to look and feel your best. It's easier and more cost-effective than ever to turn back the hands of time. By now, I hope you're feeling a little more educated and comfortable with how quick, painless, and affordable facial rejuvenation can really be. In the next chapter, we'll touch on how lasers can be a fantastic adjunct to this effort.

NINE

· · · · · · · · ·

LASERS AND LIGHT THERAPY

A wave of genius

What do CD players, supermarket checkout scanners, eye surgery, Darth Vader and facial rejuvenation have in common? They all use lasers. The technology for the use of lasers in facial rejuvenation has come a long way in the past ten years. When I started my practice, the only laser we used in facial rejuvenation was the CO_2 or carbon dioxide laser. While we still use this laser today for skin resurfacing in cases of severe sun damage, the nonsurgical platform of lasers has expanded dramatically and offers many new options for noninvasive facial rejuvenation.

WHAT EXACTLY IS A LASER?

The word *laser* is actually an acronym for Light Amplification by Simulated Emission of Radiation. Now don't let the word *radiation* scare you. Light of any type is electromagnetic radiation. Essentially, a laser is a device that emits a beam of light in which the wavelengths are very organized: the particles of light are all the same color, or wavelength, and line up perfectly with one another. Because the beam of light is so uniform, laser light can be accurately controlled and powerful.

Another class of laser-like devices are the intense pulsed light (IPL) technologies. Unlike lasers, IPL devices emit a broad spectrum of light energy that is non-coherent. Filters are used to block out unwanted wavelengths depending on the target tissue. For example, different filters may be used to treat sun spots, facial vessels, or unwanted hair. These laser-*like* devices are treated just like lasers in our practice, as they are powerful instruments and must be operated by experienced physicians, physician assistants, or advanced registered nurse practitioners.

When it comes to the use of lasers for facial rejuvenation, there are essentially two types: ablative and nonablative lasers.

Ablative lasers such as the CO_2 laser, are used for "resurfacing" the skin. Ablative lasers are more invasive in that they ablate, or remove, the top layers of damaged skin. The surface layers of the skin then heals over a period of time, resulting in a new layer of skin, thus the term *resurfacing.* While the result is dramatic, the downtime with ablative lasers can be as long as two weeks. For this reason—and because we can achieve excellent results with today's newer technology—ablative lasers are used less and less in facial rejuvenation. An ablative laser treatment is performed only by a physician and anesthesia is used. We'll discuss the CO_2 laser further in chapter twelve.

Nonablative lasers are much less invasive and work by heating up deeper layers of the skin, while leaving the surface of the skin intact. Placing the energy beneath the skin leads to collagen disruption. The body then kicks in to replace or rebuild this collagen, resulting in a gradual tightening and rejuvenation of the skin. Since the surface of the skin is not disrupted with these nonablative lasers, there is no downtime. Most of these lasers require a series of treatments to achieve optimal results. In essence, nonablative lasers achieve a slower, gradual rejuvenation over the course of six months to one year.

Let's take a closer look at some of the most effective laser systems used in our practice.

INTENSE PULSED LIGHT (IPL) LASER

You may have heard the term *photo rejuvenation.* It has nothing to do with picture-taking, rather it is a treatment for sun-damaged or "photo-aged" skin. Photo aging is the term used to describe wrinkles, brown spots and other skin damage resulting from sun exposure. An IPL treatment is a form of photo rejuvenation. It is a noninvasive laser treatment that's been around for about twenty years and the technology continues to improve each year. A "photo facial" can be performed anywhere on the body, though the face, chest and the backs of the hands and arms are the most common areas treated.

Specifically, What Concerns Does The IPL (Photo Facial) Treat?

- Brown spots (sometimes known as sun spots or age spots) and freckles resulting from sun damage anywhere on the body

- Broken and dilated capillaries (face, neck and chest)

- Redness from Rosacea

- Enlarged pore size

- Fine lines and creases

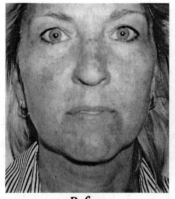 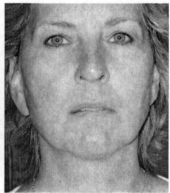

Before   *After*

An intense pulsed light (IPL) laser treatment resulted in a dramatic improvement of the pigment and texture of the skin

Is Any Preparation Required For An IPL Treatment?

Yes. There are prerequisites for an IPL treatment:

1. Avoid excessive sun exposure prior to the treatment. Excessive sun exposure can lead to redness and tanning. These additional

red and brown pigments in the skin absorb the laser light energy reducing the effectiveness of the treatment. Our newest laser, the Palomar Icon, comes with a melanin-reading device that can check for the amount of pigment in the skin and adjust the laser settings accordingly. Technology never ceases to amaze me.

2. Do not use any type of acid products (glycolic or Retin-A) on the skin for two weeks prior to treatment. Again, these more aggressive rejuvenating topical agents can induce redness in the skin, interfering with the laser treatment.

3. If you have a history of fever blisters or cold sores, you will need to be medicated before treatment with an antiviral medication.

How Is It Done?

In our office, the physician assistant administers all the IPL treatments. (Laser treatments are regulated by each state. In the state of Florida, only Advanced Registered Nurse Practitioners, Physician Assistants and Medical Doctors can do laser treatments.) A hand-held applicator is placed on the skin, and then a button is pressed to emit a short pulse of light. The newest technology in lasers provides a crystal hand piece with a chilled tip. The reds and browns in the skin absorb the flash of light energy from the laser. The applicator is then moved to the next area and another light pulse is emitted. This is repeated until the full area has been treated.

The IPL is not truly a laser, but rather a broad spectrum of noncoherent visible light energy. In other words, it is a very intense burst of light energy. Filters are used to screen out the unwanted wavelengths to target specific skin pigments like reds and browns. The effectiveness of these devices is related to some extent to the broader range of wavelengths emitted, which will target a wider range of skin pigments.

How Long Does It Take?

It takes about 45–60 minutes to treat the entire face or chest.

What's The Pain Factor?

An IPL treatment feels a bit like a rubber band striking the skin, so it stings a little. We can't use numbing creams with IPL treatments because numbing creams constrict the blood vessels and we want to be sure to get those little capillaries that are causing the redness.

Are There Any Side Effects?

Following the procedure, the face is mildly pink and puffy; the pinkness and mild swelling subside within twenty-four hours. It takes about two weeks for the broken or dilated capillaries to completely disappear. We're able to eliminate about sixty percent of the offending blood vessels with the first treatment. The treated brown spots turn darker—somewhat like the color of coffee grounds—over a two to three day period and then begin to flake off over the course of two weeks. Some patients who come to us having heard of the photo facial have the misconception that their entire face will scab over. That is not the case at all. This is a noninvasive treatment, the skin surface remains intact, and no ointments are required. Our female patients always ask if they can wear makeup after the procedure and the answer is yes.

However, makeup may not cover the brown spots as they darken before they flake off. It takes 1–2 weeks for those brown spots to fully disappear. The initial treatment eliminates about eighty percent of the offending brown spots. In our office, an IPL treatment consists of the full treatment, plus a touch up to target both the blood vessels and brown spots that weren't eliminated the first time around. Patients come in for their touch-up one month after the initial treatment. It should be noted that not all vessels and brown spots respond to the IPL treatment, but results are generally outstanding and advances in IPL technology continue to improve the efficacy of these treatments.

Is There Any Downtime?

There really is no physical downtime with the IPL treatment. There can be redness and mild swelling for up to twenty-four hours. The sun spots and vessels may be darker and more visible until they flake off, which could take up to two weeks. Final results are seen one month after the procedure.

How Long Will It Last?

The IPL is very effective and with proper skin care and avoidance of the sun, it may last for years. Of course ongoing sun exposure can lead to new or recurrent sun spots, but the IPL treatment can be repeated as needed in the future. Some patients come in every few years to address these ongoing changes.

Here's a story from Faye, a former sun worshiper who wanted to reverse her sun damage.

I Went From Using Baby Oil to Using SPF

Faye

Age: 60

I grew up in Michigan where the sun often hides behind the grey cloud cover of the Great Lakes. There were months (typically November) where we never saw the sun at all. I was a sun goddess though, and I was in the sun every possible minute, using baby oil, foil covered boards and mats to intensify the rays. During the winter, I went to the tanning booth. I travelled on Christmas and Spring breaks to Florida, Mexico or whatever warm place I could afford to go. My skin was always brown. After I retired from teaching, I moved to Florida and continued baking in the sun. There was just something about the feel of the sun on my face and body that was glorious. At the time, I actually believed my brown skin was attractive. Over the years, however, my skin had become leathery and wrinkled and I looked much older than I was. I started to realize the damage I had done.

On a routine visit, my dermatologist found an uneven spot and scheduled me to have it taken off with a biopsy. It came back pre-cancerous and although relieved it wasn't out and out cancer, I was scared to death. I knew I had logged many years in the sun and this was the beginning of a long period of payback. As much as I loved the sun, I loved my life more.

From that point forward, I decided to take care of my skin. I started having routine facials and using good skin care products. I stopped baking in the sun and used sunscreen. One of the aestheticians at Azul told me about the IPL to remove red and brown spots. In my case it was the brown blotchy spots on my face and chest that made my skin look uneven. She said I could try products to fade the brown spots, but that it would not work nearly as well as the laser and it would take a long time to get results. Products work better for those with less sun damage than I had.

Skeptical about the safety of lasers, I did a lot of research. I found that you can get burns and scarring if it is not used properly. Debbie, Dr. Flaharty's physician assistant, explained that only well-trained and licensed practitioners are supposed to use the laser, but there are unqualified people out there who are essentially breaking the law. She assured me that she had been operating the laser for eight years, and had never had a problem. She was forthcoming and honest, and I felt very comfortable. I decided to have the IPL done at Dr. Flaharty's office.

I was given a pair of goggles to wear to protect my eyes from the flash of light as the laser worked its magic. It only took about an hour, and it felt like little pinpricks or a rubber band snapping on my skin. Afterwards my skin was red. Within a few days the brown spots started to come to the surface and flake off. The whole process lasted about ten days. Because my damage was so bad, I had to go back for a second treatment. My face is now even-toned and looks great. I continue to go to Azul for my skin care, and I will probably have another procedure done. It might be the fractional laser for wrinkles, Ultherapy or a face lift with the CO_2 laser. I am not sure yet, but I know it is in my future.

My advice is to not put yourself in a position of having to correct a problem. Use sunscreen and if you want to be tan, get the spray on tan, or use self-tanning products or bronzer. If you have damage from the sun, start to reverse it now.

LASER HAIR REMOVAL

Laser hair removal has been a very effective and popular treatment to assist patients in reducing unwanted hair anywhere on the body. Hair removal requires a series of 6–8 treatments, 2 weeks to 2 months apart, depending on the area treated. (Hair grows in cycles. We try to hit every cycle, thus the multiple treatments.) The best candidates for laser hair removal are people with dark, coarse hair. The hair must have pigment to respond to the laser and coarse hair responds better than fine hair. Black and brown hair responds the best, grey hair slightly less effectively, and fine light hair (peach fuzz on the face) responds poorly.

Is Any Preparation Required?

Yes, you must shave the area to be treated.

How Is It Done?

Laser hair removal is done with a contact hand piece. The light energy is delivered to the skin in pulses. The energy is absorbed by the pigment in the hair follicle destroying the bulb. Only active, growing hairs respond to the laser and as such, a series of treatments is required. Not every hair will be eliminated by laser hair removal, however, it is a very effective solution to substantially reduce unwanted hair in good candidates.

How Long Does It Take?

Each treatment takes 10–60 minutes, depending on the area being treated.

What's the Pain Factor?

The discomfort depends on the area being treated, with the bikini line and upper lip being the most uncomfortable. Our patients generally rate the most intense discomfort as moderate. Newer technology with a "cool tip" hand piece is faster and less painful than previous lasers.

Are There Any Side Effects?

The common side effects include some redness and swelling at the treatment site that can last up to twenty-four hours.

Is There Any Downtime?

Immediately after your treatment, you should avoid swimming pools, hot tubs and strenuous activity resulting in perspiration for twenty-four hours.

How Long Will It Last?

The hair follicles that are destroyed are gone for good, but remember, about ten percent of the hair will not be eliminated. Hair that regrows is fine and lighter than the hair removed.

FRACTIONAL LASER

One of the new treatment concepts in laser skin rejuvenation is called fractional technology. There are a number of fractional lasers now on the market, and they can be either ablative (removing the skin) or nonablative (leaving the skin intact.) The driving force in the development of fractional laser systems was an attempt to achieve results similar to fully-ablative CO_2 laser resurfacing, while reducing the downtime and potential complications. Instead of removing the entire surface of the skin—as is the case with the CO_2 laser—the ablative fractional laser selectively removes tiny spots of skin in a checkerboard pattern. The intervening skin is left intact and serves as a source for skin cells to generate new skin over the ablated columns. Fractional ablative laser resurfacing still has some downtime, but heals much faster than fully-ablative resurfacing. Topical ointments are indicated and patients must avoid the sun for 7–10 days. Fully ablative resurfacing usually requires two weeks of healing time but generally yields much better results in terms of wrinkle reduction and elimination of sun damaged skin. In my opinion, the ablative fractional lasers have been disappointing: they are uncomfortable, have substantial downtime, and do not achieve the same level of improvement as the fully-ablative CO_2 laser.

The nonablative fractional laser systems, on the other hand, are proving to be a very useful office-based laser system for noninvasive skin tightening. We use the Palomar 1540 which delivers a grid of pulses "beneath" the skin. This creates disruption of collagen in columns while keeping the skin surface intact. This means there is no downtime or need for ointment as the skin surface is not removed. All these lasers essentially work the same way in that they create an injury in the skin. Remarkably, the body's healing response is what creates the rejuvenation. In the case of the nonablative fractional laser, the stimulation of new collagen under the skin will tighten the skin gradually, reducing wrinkles. Because the improvement occurs more gradually, a series of four treatments, each separated by one month, is required. Total improvement continues for up to six months after the last treatment.

What Concerns Can It Treat?

- Overall facial wrinkles

- Grainy skin texture, including "orange-peel" textured skin

- Crow's feet

- Vertical lines around the mouth

- Crepey skin in the cheek area

- Surgical scars

- Acne scars

- Stretch marks on the body

Is Any Preparation Required?

This treatment is beneath the skin, so there is no concern about acid products or suntan. If you have a history of fever blisters or cold sores however, you will need to take an antiviral medication before being treated. No other special preparation is needed.

How Is It Done?

Numbing cream is applied for thirty minutes prior to the treatment to minimize any discomfort. Unlike the IPL treatment, these topical numbing creams do not adversely affect the fractional laser results. As with the IPL treatment, the person administering the treatment places a hand-held applicator on the skin, and then presses a button to emit a pulse of fractional energy. The applicator is then moved to the next area and another pulse is delivered. This is repeated until the full area has been treated.

How Long Does It Take?

Numbing time is approximately thirty minutes. The treatment itself takes around twenty minutes.

What's The Pain Factor?

There is mild discomfort associated with the fractional laser; we do use numbing cream. We've done hundreds of fractional laser treatments and have never had a patient who couldn't tolerate the discomfort.

Are There Any Side Effects?

Immediately following the treatment, the face is moderately pink. Swelling is mild and actually looks good because it fills in all the nooks and crannies. The pinkness subsides in a few hours and the mild swelling subsides over several days. Some patients are disappointed when the swelling goes away and some of the lines and creases return.

What Is The Downtime?

There really is no downtime with the fractional laser, and this is one of its main advantages.

How Long Before The Full Effect Is Realized?

Because the nonablative fractional laser treatments gradually stimulate collagen formation, it takes 6–9 months following the last procedure in the series before you will enjoy the full result. In other words, from start to finish, you're looking at one year. With this treatment, you will enjoy a 50–75 percent reduction in fine lines and wrinkles.

Can The Fractional Laser Be Combined With Botox And/Or Fillers?

Most fillers are placed a little deeper into the dermis (or beneath the skin) than the layer of skin targeted by the fractional or IPL lasers, and there is no evidence to suggest that lasers will "melt" fillers. However, we prefer to be safe and recommend waiting one month after the placement of fillers to perform the laser treatment. Conversely, we need to wait only a few days after the lasers to perform fillers or Botox, just long enough for the swelling to subside.

How Long Will It Last?

We recommend a touch up once each year to continue to stimulate collagen for the full face treatments. The first touch up is done twelve months after your last treatment. Scar treatment can be permanent once the collagen grows in, especially if it's a small scar. Touch ups for scars are recommended based on individual patient needs.

A Note About Equipment

The laser machine we use at Azul Cosmetic Surgery and Medical Spa is manufactured by Palomar. The same machine—with different hand pieces—is used for IPL treatments, the nonablative fractional laser, and laser hair removal. We've used Palomar equipment for more than twenty years and are very happy with the results it produces for our patients. Less than a year ago, I upgraded to the state of the art Palomar Icon™ Aesthetic System. At Azul, we keep up with the latest technology advancements in order to offer the best possible results for our patients. When you do your homework, you may want to inquire so you can be certain the doctor you're considering is using state-of-the-art equipment. With the rate of advancement in technology, the latest equipment can make a difference.

Laser technology is constantly becoming more and more advanced, thus allowing us to leverage technology to produce outstanding results for our patients—at a fraction of the cost of the more invasive surgeries in decades past. Whether therapies are combined or utilized on their own, patients are constantly bowled over by both the ease of treatment and astonishing results new technologies help the practitioner achieve. In chapter ten, we'll continue to look at more technologies available to reach your goals. Our patient, Robert, was very excited to see what technology could do for him.

Thanks to Technology, My Scars Are Barely Visible

Robert

Age: 42

I'm in the media, and looks are important for my job. I got into a cycling accident and had very deep cuts on my forehead. Although I had a plastic surgeon sew me up, I still had visible scars, which bothered me and I was very self-conscious about them. (Guys can't get away with looking rugged in the media these days.) I could hide the redness with makeup, but I couldn't hide the sunken-in scar lines. A friend of mine—whose girlfriend had recently had laser treatments for acne scarring—suggested I see Dr. Flaharty for my scars.

I went to see Dr. Flaharty and he was great. We bonded immediately, as he is a cyclist too. We swapped biking stories and I was immediately comfortable. He told me not to worry that he would have me in tip-top shape and nobody would be able to see my scars after we were done. The plan was to do a combination of lasers and fillers. The laser stimulates collagen which would eventually help fill in the scars, but in the meantime he would inject fillers to plump out the depression. His nurse put numbing cream on the areas to be treated with the laser, and Dr. Flaharty walked with me to the other side of the clinic where the laser room is located.

Debbie worked me into her schedule for my first laser treatment, as I was very eager to get started. It only took about fifteen minutes. Afterwards, the scars and area around them were really red, but that subsided in about twenty-four hours. Dr. Flaharty told me to come back in a week for fillers in the scar depressions, which I did. My scars already looked much better and with TV studio make up, you couldn't tell at all.

I had to go back three more times for laser sessions, and I got two additional treatments of filler. Today my scars are barely noticeable. I'm grateful that technology could virtually erase my scars.

TEN

· · · · · · · · · ·

ULTHERAPY

Defying gravity

The search for low-impact ways to rejuvenate the face is ongoing. The latest technology in this field is a tissue-tightening treatment called Ultherapy, an exciting technology and the newest noninvasive facial rejuvenation addition to our office. Ultherapy lifts and tightens the face and neck and involves:

- No downtime

- No incisions

- No preparation

Ultherapy is not a light-based laser. Rather, it uses ultrasound energy. You may have heard of, or perhaps experienced, an "ultrasound test." Ultrasound-based diagnostic imaging has been used in the medical world for years and one of the more common uses of ultrasound is imaging for pregnant women. Ultrasound is acoustic or sound energy—above the range of human hearing— in the form of waves. This new technology uses focused ultrasound energy delivered to the deeper layers of the face beneath the skin to tighten and lift. The figure below shows where Ultherapy energy is focused as opposed to lasers.

Over the years, our patients have consistently inquired about nonsurgical options for lifting and tightening. Ultherapy is the first FDA approved nonsurgical technology to lift the face. Although the results achieved with Ultherapy do not rival those of a brow lift, face lift or neck lift, the results can be quite dramatic which is impressive for a one-time only noninvasive, no downtime procedure.

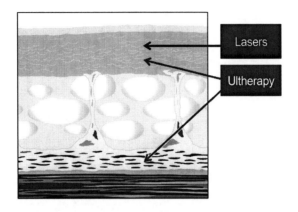

Lasers work at the top layers of the skin. Ultherapy targets deeper tissues to lift and tighten the face, while firming and toning the skin.

WHAT CONCERNS DOES ULTHERAPY TREAT?

1. Drooping eyelid

2. Drooping brow

3. Lower face laxity

4. Jowling

5. Neck laxity

How Does Ultherapy Work To Lift And Tighten?

The high-frequency sound waves produced by the Ultherapy machine target the deeper suspensory layers of the face called the superficial musculoaponeurotic system, or "SMAS" for short. The SMAS layer is the main suspensory layer of the face, which is tightened and lifted during face and neck lift surgery. With the aid of the visible ultrasound screen, the focused ultrasound energy is delivered into the SMAS layer in rows, creating instant tightening and setting off a cascade of new collagen formation, which will result in further tightening and lifting of the tissues. Heating these layers of tissue causes the tissue to bind more closely. There is shrinkage of tissue without cutting, lifting or suturing. In addition, the ultrasound energy stimulates your body's own skin-plumping system: collagen. New collagen is produced over a 3–4 month period. The result is a firming, tightening and lifting of the skin. Ultherapy sets a regenerative process in motion, gradually rejuvenating your face from the inside out.

Who Is The Ideal Candidate For Ultherapy?

While patients of all ages are excited by the Ultherapy technology, the best results are seen on younger patients, say up to age fifty-five, or patients up to age sixty who do not have a lot of neck sagging. The ideal candidates for Ultherapy are men and women with mild skin laxity: those who are not quite ready for a face lift. Ultherapy is also a good choice for patients who have had a face lift in the past and are starting to experience some laxity or stretching of the tissues.

There will always be patients who do not want surgery and of course, Ultherapy is an option for them, as long as they know what to expect. While the results with Ultherapy can be impressive for a noninvasive procedure, surgery remains the gold standard for lifting, firming and tightening. Even though the result with Ultherapy will not be as dramatic as with surgery, for a forty-five minute, no-downtime procedure, the result can be quite remarkable. Of course, results will vary from patient to patient. The statistics suggest that eighty-five percent of Ultherapy patients notice appreciable firming and tightening of the facial tissues treated. This means that fifteen percent of patients may not see much noticeable tightening with one treatment and may require a second treatment.

Is Any Preparation Required?

There is no preparation required for an Ultherapy treatment.

How Is It Done?

In our office, both our medical aesthetician and our physician assistant perform the Ultherapy procedure. Like all Ultherapy practitioners, they have gone through extensive, hands-on training. After cleansing your skin, the practitioner applies an ultrasound gel to the areas to be treated. The hand piece from the Ultherapy machine is then placed on the skin and the ultrasound energy is emitted with the push of a button. The hand piece is then moved to the next area, until the entire area has been treated.

How Long Does It Take?

The entire procedure takes 1–2 hours depending on whether the full face, or just the lower face is being treated.

What's The Pain Factor?

There is some discomfort with the Ultherapy treatment, though it is temporary (only during the treatment) and mild to moderate in intensity. We manage potential discomfort by giving our patients a pain medication, or in some cases, a pain medication cocktail which includes the pain medication and an anti-anxiety medication. Patients who take sedating pain medications need someone to drive them home.

What Are The Side Effects?

Your skin may appear a bit flushed immediately after the treatment, but redness disappears within a few hours. You may have slight swelling for a few days or tingling and tenderness to the touch.

Is There Any Downtime?

There is no downtime with Ultherapy. You may resume life as normal as soon as you leave our office.

How Long Before The Full Effect Is Realized?

You may enjoy a small amount of tightening immediately with Ultherapy, though new collagen will continue to form over the course of 2–3 months, and sometimes up to four months. We advise our patients that the full effect of Ultherapy will not be seen for four months.

Can Ultherapy Be Combined With Botox And/Or Fillers?

Ultherapy can be combined with the injectables, but we do not do Ultherapy, fillers and Botox all at the same time. Ultherapy targets a deeper layer of the face, and it is quite possible that the fillers could be affected during Ultherapy treatment. Therefore, we recommend having Ultherapy first and then following up with fillers a week later. Alternatively, after fillers, we recommend patients wait six weeks before having the Ultherapy treatment so the fillers are completely settled in and integrated.

There are no restrictions on concurrent use of Botox and Ultherapy. In fact, many physicians will do the Botox immediately after Ultherapy, while others wait 1–2 weeks. At Azul, we prefer to wait 1–2 weeks after Ultherapy before we administer Botox.

How Long Will It Last?

Ultherapy is a new technology, so the studies go back only a few years. Although initially touted to last eighteen months, the company is now reporting good results lasting up to two years. Like all technologies, the results will vary. Some of our patients have achieved dramatic results which seem to hold up very well over time, while others may demonstrate only mild improvement. Although it is considered a one-time treatment, Ultherapy can be repeated, either at six months (to achieve further improvement) or after a few years as the effects begin to fade. Lisa loves the result of her Ultherapy treatment.

I Staved Off Surgery For a Few Years With Ultherapy

Lisa

Age: 50

When it comes to my health and appearance, I've been a long-time believer in maintenance. Over the past nine years I've maintained my appearance with the help of injectables (Botox, Restylane, and Juvederm.) However, in the last few years I've noticed the familiar descent of my jaw line and lower chin, a family trait. I decided to ask Dr. Flaharty—who does my Botox and fillers—about my options. I was thinking surgery, but Dr. Flaharty said I would be a good candidate for Ultherapy. I loved the fact that there is no downtime so I did it.

It was an in-office procedure and only took about an hour. The day after, I had a little tenderness to the touch along my jawline and when I turned my head. Three days later, there was a little yellowing along my jawline, which I was able to hide with makeup.

I was told that results would be seen in about four months, but my husband noticed improvement in about forty-five days. I agreed. I noticed the jowl was lifting. It has been five months now and I'm very pleased with the results. My friends have also noticed the results and some have decided to get Ultherapy as well. I feel that for a noninvasive, no-downtime, in-office treatment, I got just the results I was looking for. I staved off the surgical procedure a few more years.

Today's skilled cosmetic surgeons are at the forefront of medical research, clinical practice, and nonsurgical innovations that improve the health, vitality and beauty of the skin. In the next chapter, we'll talk about how surgery remains a superior option for many men and women in the quest to look as energetic and vital as they feel, at any age.

ELEVEN

· · · · · · · · · · · · ·

SURGERY

The gold standard

Although advances in noninvasive and minimally invasive procedures have been dramatic in recent years, there are certain aspects of facial rejuvenation that can be achieved only with surgery. Surgery is at the apex of the pyramid, as it often represents a natural progression up the pyramid with age. Surgical rejuvenation also represents the pinnacle of what we do as surgeons. Surgical rejuvenation—always my true passion as a surgeon—is often a once-in-a-lifetime event for patients. My favorite time of the week is the quiet, focused atmosphere of the operating room. Spending a few hours rejuvenating a face—turning back the hands of time perhaps ten or twenty years—is challenging and meaningful work and incredibly rewarding both for me and my patients. The "unveiling" the day after surgery when we remove the dressings in our office is equally exciting as the patient gets to see their new face for the first time. The subsequent "blossoming" over the next few weeks as the new face settles into final shape is a powerful and wonderful metamorphosis. Although there are more and more noninvasive and minimally invasive techniques to rejuvenate the face, there is nothing more powerful than panfacial rejuvenation where the entire face is rejuvenated in a single procedure resulting in a beautiful, harmonious transformation back in time.

The popularity of facial cosmetic surgery has increased dramatically in the past two decades. Better understanding of facial anatomy, technological advances, and improved anesthetic techniques have all led to shorter operating times, more natural-looking results, and less post-surgery downtime. According to Jeffrey M. Kenkel, MD, President of the American Society for Aesthetic Plastic Surgery, "Since 1997, the interest in and demand for cosmetic plastic surgery has risen exponentially." Even with all the advances in nonsurgical facial rejuvenation, the face lift remains the ultimate in facial rejuvenation.

Prior to surgery, every patient is scheduled for a "pre-op visit" in the office. Typically this pre-op appointment is scheduled two weeks prior to your surgical procedure. The timing of this appointment is somewhat flexible depending on the patient's needs; we have many patients who come to Florida from other parts of the country. During your pre-op appointment, we review the specifics of your procedure, answer any and all questions you may have, provide you with pre and post-surgery instructions, and give you any necessary prescriptions. Anyone over the age of fifty must have an EKG prior to surgery if their procedure will be two hours or longer. No additional medical clearance is necessary unless the patient has a chronic disease that would be affected by anesthesia. We also take your "before photos" during this visit.

All of our surgeries are performed at a nationally certified surgical center. We offer a private pre and post-surgical room at the center exclusively for our cosmetic surgery patients. Only one person at a time is accommodated in this room. The surgical center staff readies patients for surgery and manages their recovery after the surgery. We have a consistent surgical team of dedicated professionals who are committed to making your experience as pleasant as possible.

The anesthesia—an IV sedation, similar to the anesthesia you would have for a colonoscopy—is the same for all surgical procedures. The anesthesia is administered by a certified nurse anesthetist who is at your side during the entire procedure. We also have board certified anesthesiologists on staff who are on site for all surgical procedures; the highest level of patient safety is paramount. After the procedure, surgical patients typically spend 30–60 minutes in recovery and are fairly awake by the time they leave for home.

WHAT ARE THE SURGICAL PROCEDURES FOR FACIAL REJUVENATION?

There are eight main facial surgical procedures that address the aging face:

1. Eyelid surgery (Blepharoplasty)

2. Brow lift (typically endoscopic brow lift)

3. Face lift (Rhytidectomy)

4. Neck lift

5. Fat transfer

6. Chin augmentation

7. CO_2 laser resurfacing

8. Dermabrasion

Is Any Preparation Required For Surgical Facial Rejuvenation?

The preparation for all facial surgical procedures is the same, and mostly revolves around taking precautions to reduce bleeding during surgery. For one week prior to surgery, you must avoid alcohol and any drugs or herbals that may increase bleeding. These include aspirin, blood thinners—including fish oils and botanicals—and anti-inflammatory drugs of any type. During those seven days prior to surgery, we recommend to our patients that they eat fresh pineapple to help with bleeding.

Who Is The Ideal Candidate For Surgical Facial Rejuvenation?

The ideal surgical candidate is a nonsmoker in good health with a positive attitude. Surgical candidates should be contemplating surgery for the right reasons and have reasonable expectations regarding their outcome.

How Long Do Surgical Procedures Last?

For most patients, surgical facial rejuvenation procedures are a once-in-a-lifetime event, and therefore, a one-time expense. Depending on the procedure, many patients continue to come to the office for treatments (such as skin care, Botox, fillers, and in-office lasers) that will help maintain the wonderful result of their surgical procedure. As we are living longer and staying healthier, some patients will come back ten, fifteen, or twenty years after the initial procedure to discuss further surgery. These secondary procedures are often very different than the primary surgery, due to ongoing aging changes and the evolution of new techniques.

Before we delve into the particulars of each of the surgical facial rejuvenation procedures, I'd like to share Karen's story with you.

My Mother Had Plastic Surgery, So I Always Knew I Would, Too

Karen

Age: 58

I'm a salesperson. There's an unspoken salesperson mentality that says anyone in sales needs to look the part: women in sales get their hair and nails done; they wear nice clothes, and always have a gorgeous handbag. Ever since getting into sales I've followed this unspoken protocol.

Growing up I had acne, so I've always had a complex that I wasn't attractive. Then, ten years ago, I got divorced. My mother had two plastic surgery procedures: a face lift in her mid-fifties and another one in her early seventies, so it was always in the back of my mind that I would do something. The first thing I did was to have eyelid surgery. I also got hair extensions around the same time. People started telling me I looked younger.

About six years later, I decided I wanted something more. I had moved to the west coast of Florida and was in a new job. I was out to dinner with a friend, and when I told her she looked great, she told me she'd had a face lift with Dr. Flaharty. I called and scheduled a consultation with him. I didn't think I was ready for a face lift, but I wanted something. I ended up having Dr. Flaharty's Liquid Face Lift, though I did inquire about a surgical face lift. A few months later, I went to one of Dr. Flaharty's seminars and that's when I decided to have a face lift. Two weeks after the seminar, I scheduled my surgery for seven months later, which was the end of August.

On the day of the surgery, I was really nervous. My mom went with me and was in the waiting room. I had to keep in my mind that I trusted my doctor, but I kept thinking, "what if they make a mistake?" I realized I was actually more afraid of the anesthesia than the actual surgery. Everyone at the surgery center was super. I think they were all hired, not only because they're great at what they do, but because they're just really nice people. They completely put me at ease and explained everything. I got to talk with the anesthesiologist before the surgery. It ended up being a very pleasant experience.

I took ten days off. For me, sleeping on my back was the hardest part of the recovery. I never took any pain medication. For some reason, day three was my worst day. The only people who knew I was having surgery were my kids and of course, my mom. When I went back to work after ten days, I still had a little bit of bruising. For the most part, I was able to cover it up with makeup. If anyone asked, I told them I was in a minor car accident and the airbag went off.

I'm really happy with the result. People don't believe I'm fifty-eight. I had gone into surgery with a photo of myself when I was fifteen. I think I look like I did when I was in my twenties.

There are a number of things that surprised me. They give you fifty pages to read, but I never did get to read it all. If I had, perhaps I wouldn't have been surprised, so I would tell others to ask questions and know what to expect. For example, they cut into the hairline. There are a couple places where my hair didn't grow back. I also had some bleeding behind my ears initially. The first couple of nights I didn't sleep because I can't sleep on my back, but then they prescribed Ambien for me. You can't wash your hair with regular shampoo: you have to use baby shampoo and I always felt like my hair was greasy. You can't do any heavy exercise. For a while, when I would ride my bike, it was uncomfortable wearing my helmet.

My advice to others: if you feel like you want to look younger, go for it. I can tell you that having a C-Section was ten times worse! Just be sure to have someone with you for the first couple of days.

EYELID SURGERY (BLEPHAROPLASTY)

Sometimes called an eyelid lift, eyelid surgery is often the first foray into any type of facial cosmetic surgery. Eyelids are very delicate and are often the first area to show signs of aging. This may include heaviness and drooping of the upper eyelid, bulging fat in the upper and lower eyelids, loose skin around the eyes, and wrinkles. Technically called blepharoplasty, eyelid surgery can improve the appearance of the upper eyelids, the lower eyelids, or both. Upper eyelid surgery corrects a drooping eyelid, which can not only cause the individual to appear tired and older, but can also impair vision. Upper eyelid surgery can also remove eyelid puffiness (due to excess fat,) and loose skin and wrinkles.

Lower eyelid surgery is performed for one of three reasons: to eliminate bags under the eyes due to excessive fat, to remove or tighten excess skin and wrinkles under the eye, and to correct a drooping lower lid. (When the lower eyelid droops, it shows the whites of the eyes below the iris.) In recent years it has also become very common to use HA fillers at the time of eyelid surgery to fill in the dark circles or hollows that occur under the lower eyelids. This can also be performed with fat if fat transfer is to be performed. (We'll talk about fat transfer later in this chapter.) Eyelid surgery results in a rested, younger, and more alert look.

How Is Eyelid Surgery Done?

Many factors are taken into account with eyelid surgery, including the amount of excess fat and skin, and the position of the eyebrows. Measurements of the eyelid are taken using a special instrument. I take these measurements twice: before my patient goes into the operating room and then again in the operating room. Removing just the right amount of skin is crucial to the success of upper eyelid surgery. Knowing how much to remove comes both from experience and from taking measurements. For upper eyelid surgery, an incision is made in the natural crease of the eyelid. Any excess skin and/or fatty tissue is removed through this incision. In recent years I have tended toward preserving the fat around the eye as much as possible to avoid future hollowness. Of course, if the fat is excessive and creating unattractive bulges around the eyes, it can be trimmed or sculpted to the desired contour.

For the lower eyelids, surgery is performed differently, depending on the problem. If the concern is loose skin with fine wrinkles, the incision is made directly under the lower eyelashes. The skin is smoothed and the excess skin is removed. If the problem is fat under eyes, the incision is made inside the eyelid, and the fat removed. We also use chemical peels and laser peels to tighten and smooth out lower eyelid wrinkles when necessary. In addition, we often use an HA filler in the dark circles or hollows under the lower eyelids at the time of surgery. Removing these dark circles really improves the cosmetic result in lower eyelid surgery.

Many insurance plans cover upper eyelid surgery if the excess skin is affecting vision. In order to determine if upper eyelid surgery will be covered by insurance, we do very specific testing called "visual fields" that measures just how much your eyelids may be interfering with your vision. This information gets submitted to your insurance company and a determination of coverage is made.

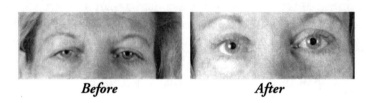

Before   *After*

This patient's eyes are more open—and the shape of the lids is more youthful—following eyelid surgery (blepharoplasty.)

How Long Does The Surgery Take?

Eyelid surgery generally takes 30–60 minutes, depending on the extent of surgery.

What Is The Pain Factor?

The good news is that there really is minimal discomfort associated with eyelid surgery. Patients may notice mild tenderness or sensitivity around the eyes for a few weeks.

Are There Any Side Effects?

The eyelids swell easily because the skin is very thin and loose. The risk of swelling and bruising is significant with eyelid surgery and we strongly recommend frequent ice packs immediately after surgery. Applying ice packs intermittently for the first forty-eight hours will help reduce the swelling and bruising. Some patients prefer to use ice intermittently for the first week until most of the swelling has resolved.

What Is The Healing Process?

Pain with eyelid surgery is minimal, but the risk of swelling is real. Once you're settled back at home after eyelid surgery (upper, lower, or both) you'll apply ice every hour for fifteen minutes for the rest of the day. Beginning the day following eyelid surgery, ice is applied 4–6 times each day for forty-eight hours. Antibiotic ointment is applied over the stitches every night at bedtime. Care must be taken with sleeping positions, and this can be the biggest challenge of eyelid surgery. It is important to sleep slightly elevated with the back of the head on the pillow for the first three nights. Stitches are removed in our office six days after surgery. It can take up to two weeks—and sometimes longer—for most of the swelling and bruising to disappear. We ask patients to be gentle with the eyelid area: no rubbing or scrubbing for two weeks, and no strenuous exercise for two weeks. Walking or riding a stationary bike is permitted.

How Long Before The Full Effect Is Realized?

You will see an immediate improvement with eyelid surgery, but the cosmetic benefit is best appreciated once the swelling and bruising have subsided over the course of two weeks. Some patients may have visible swelling or discoloration for 4–6 weeks.

Shannon, a professional athlete, had an eyelid lift at age 41.

As A Professional Athlete, I Need to Look and Feel My Best

Shannon

Age: 41

I compete in figure competitions, in the International Federation of Body Building figure division. It's a pretty big sport. I'd been competing at the national level for two years. When I looked at myself in pictures, I noticed that my eyelids were beginning to droop, the left one more than the right. It bothered me a little, but not enough to do anything about it. Then last year I turned pro. When I looked at my new stage photos, all I saw was my eye: it looked half shut. That was it. I decided to do something about it.

I knew Dr. Flaharty because a couple of years ago, I started going to his medical aesthetician for skin care. Because I felt good about everyone in his office, I decided to go to him for consultation for eyelid surgery. I made the decision right away to have Dr. Flaharty do the surgery. The day of the surgery I was petrified. All I could think was, "What if I don't look right." The staff at the surgery center was great. They answered all my questions and helped me to relax. Everyone in Dr. Flaharty's office really cares. Dr. Flaharty himself called me the day after the surgery to check on me.

I was a very compliant patient and diligent about following instructions for post-surgery. The first two days I sat around on the couch and used my ice packs. I only missed two days of work. In fact, I went back to work on Friday, and then went to a big affair on Sunday. No one knew I'd had eyelid surgery until I pointed it out, and I still had the stitches in then. I had minimum bruising.

I'm thrilled with the results. My advice to others is definitely to get eyelid surgery if you're self-conscious about your eyelids.

ENDOSCOPIC BROW LIFT

Many patients come in for consultations regarding eyelid surgery only to discover that their main problem is a droopy forehead. (A brow lift and a forehead lift are the same thing.) The advent of endoscopic brow lifts in the early 1990s turned out to be a very important advance in facial cosmetic surgery. Gone are the days of large forehead incisions. The endoscopic brow lift is the most current technique, and the one I use most often. In my opinion, the endoscopic brow lift is one of the biggest advances in the surgical rejuvenation of the face. Advantages of using the endoscope (an instrument that is used to visualize under the skin) include smaller incisions, less bruising and quicker recovery. An endoscopic brow lift can reposition a low or sagging brow, correct much of the heavy skin of the upper eyelid, smooth out the lines that develop across the forehead, minimize frown lines between the eyebrows, and correct wrinkles at the outer corners of the eyelids. Many patients enjoy a lifting of the eyelids as a benefit of the brow lift, though a brow lift doesn't always negate the need for eyelid surgery. Often, brow lift and eyelid surgeries are combined. It all depends on the needs of the individual. According to the American Society of Plastic Surgeons (ASPS), the number of brow lifts performed in the United States has risen 172 percent since 1992.[10] This increase in frequency of brow lifts is likely related to the new endoscopic approach to brow lifting which is quicker, safer, and more effective—with less risk of swelling, bruising, and numbness—than the older open brow lift techniques.

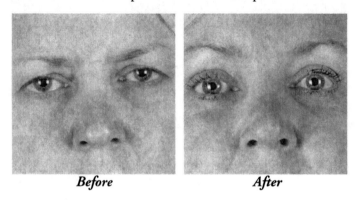

Before   *After*

A brow lift alone can often improve a patient's expression, and the appearance of the eyelids.

How Is The Brow Lift Done?

We make four very tiny incisions in the hair of the scalp. Through these little incisions, we use our delicate instruments to release and elevate the tissues of the forehead, upper eyelids, and lateral eyelid areas. Once reshaped to the position we desire, the brow (both the skin and the underlying tissue) is held in place with endotines. (The endotine is a medical device that is superior to sutures for holding the lifted brow in place while it heals. Forehead endotines are made of the same material as dissolvable sutures and are eventually absorbed into the body.) This is an elegant procedure because we can do it through tiny incisions even your hairdresser can't find. In addition, the endotine fixation of the brow allows a very accurate control over the height and contour of the brow.

How Long Does the Surgery Take?

The total time for the endoscopic brow lift is approximately one hour.

What Is the Pain Factor?

After the brow lift, some patients complain of a headache that may last 24–48 hours. In addition, the skin over the endotines will be tender to the touch for several weeks. Sensitivity in the area of the endotines—when washing and brushing your hair—may last 2–3 months.

Are There Any Side Effects?

The incisions are closed with delicate, dissolvable sutures and heal very quickly. Swelling and bruising can occur around the eyelids, though is generally mild. Some patients will feel some numbness in the forehead which can last anywhere from two weeks to a few months.

What Is The Healing Process?

The swelling and bruising around the eyes can last for a few weeks. The day after surgery, patients can wash their hair, but we encourage all our patients to be gentle for a few months when washing their hair. We also ask patients to be gentle with the brow and forehead areas: no rubbing or scrubbing for two weeks, and no strenuous exercise for two weeks. Walking or riding a stationary bike is permitted. Most patients return to light activity within 2–3 days, and go back to work in a week.

How Long Before The Full Effect Is Realized?

You will see the result of your brow lift immediately, though there may be some swelling that will subside within two weeks. Final results are visible within a few months.

FACE LIFT AND NECK LIFT

One of the common misconceptions about a face lift is that it deals with the entire face. It does not. A face lift is for the lower face only. A face lift is ideal for someone with a lot of loose skin and fat in the lower part of the face. The typical face lift patient is usually at least fifty years old. I'll review both the face lift and the neck lift in this section—because more often than not—these two procedures are performed together.

What Exactly Is A Face Lift And How Is It Done?

A face lift is a procedure that involves tightening the loose soft tissue structures of the lower face and neck. Discreet incisions are made in the hairline and in the natural creases around the ears. A delicate skin flap is developed to reveal the deeper suspensory structure of the face, (the SMAS, which is the same layer targeted in Ultherapy.) This deeper suspensory layer can be lifted and tightened, which lifts the lower face and neck. It is important to tighten at this deep level because it gives the most complete and longest-lasting face lift. The skin is also lifted and tightened over the newly tightened muscle, and put back in a *natural way*, avoiding the pulled appearance which can be a tell-tale sign of a face lift. Good technique is paramount for natural results.

The neck lift is almost always incorporated in a face lift to achieve the most complete and natural rejuvenation of the lower face and neck. Liposuction of the lower face and neck is also commonly performed with this procedure to reduce unwanted fat from the neck, improving the jawline and neck contour.

How Long Does The Surgery Take?

A face and neck lift procedure takes roughly two hours, but is often combined with other procedures such as an endoscopic brow lift, eyelid surgery, or fat transfer which can add an additional 1–2 hours to the procedure.

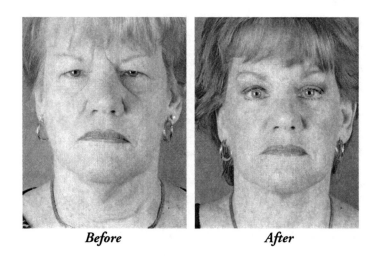

Before   *After*

Notice the youthful appearance this patient achieves after an endoscopic brow lift, and a face and neck lift.

What's The Pain Factor?

One of the most frequently asked questions about face lifts—and all cosmetic surgery for that matter—is, "Will it hurt?" Typically patients are pleasantly surprised to learn that face lifts are generally not painful. Patients wear a soft head wrap the first evening to hold all the tissues in place and reduce the risk of swelling and bruising. This dressing is removed the next morning in the office. Patients will experience some tightness, numbness and soreness that gradually resolve over several weeks to months. Although we give our patients a prescription for narcotic pain medication, most use these meds only for the first few days and then they use ibuprofen or other over-the-counter pain pills.

What Are The Side Effects?

The typical side effects with surgery include swelling and bruising, though it is different for each individual. Everyone experiences temporary numbness in front of the ears due to the manipulation of the skin in the lower face and neck lift. The numbness will gradually resolve over several months. Some patients may note areas of numbness for up to a year.

What Is The Healing Process?

We recommend eating soft foods the first few days to avoid excessive chewing. We also ask patients to be gentle with the face: no rubbing or scrubbing for two weeks, and no strenuous exercise for two weeks. Walking or riding a stationary bike is permitted. You can wash your hair the day after surgery, being careful not to disrupt the incisions. Our tissues heal very rapidly and are generally very stable by two weeks. An elastic support band is used in some cases to provide gentle support for the face and neck in the first week.

How Long Before The Full Effect Is Realized?

Patients come to the office at one and two weeks post-surgery, then again three months after surgery. It's fair to say that most patients look fairly normal approximately two weeks after surgery although some can experience visible swelling and bruising for 4–6 weeks. Some patients lay low for two weeks while others are back to work or out to dinner within a week. Makeup can be helpful in assisting the patient's return to normal activities.

THE MINI-LIFT OR "S-LIFT"

For those men and women who don't need a full face lift, we have a "lower impact" version of the face lift. It's called the mini-lift, or S-Lift. Advantages of the mini-lift include smaller incisions, less downtime, less bruising and less overall trauma. The incisions for the mini-lift are about half the length of traditional face lift incisions. Nonetheless, the mini-lift provides significant, lasting results for properly-selected patients. It will reduce jowls, tighten neck skin, and narrow and refine the lower face, restoring its proper proportion in relation to the upper face. The only way to know which type of face lift is the right one for you is to have a consultation. Although mini-lifts sound attractive, they are best suited for younger patients with early stages of laxity. They are limited in their ability to tighten and rejuvenate the neck, and therefore, are not commonly recommended for most face lift candidates. Sharon, however, was the perfect candidate for a mini-lift.

I Was Turning 50 and Wanted To "Do Something"

Sharon

Age: 61

When I was nearing fifty, I looked in the mirror one day and realized I didn't love what I saw. I have really big eyes, but my eyelids were hooded and I felt as though I looked tired all the time. I wanted a more youthful appearance. I knew I wanted something done, but I wasn't sure what. I was certain I did not want a face lift. I assumed what I needed was eyelid surgery.

I got excited just thinking about it and started asking lots of questions of friends who'd had some work done: who was their doctor? Would they recommend him or her? Were they happy with what they had done? How was the recovery? I talked to lots of friends up north who had things done. I had one really good friend who overdid it. I had another friend who just looked younger and fresher. They're both seventy-five now and still look good.

I decided to take it a step further and consult with different doctors. I made appointments for consultations with doctors who do faces and nothing else. I've seen women with really bad plastic surgery; it looks awful and unnatural and I wanted no part of that, so it was important to me that I find a facial plastic surgeon as opposed to a general plastic surgeon. I went to three doctors in total. When I met with Dr. Flaharty, I knew I could trust him with my face: he was very calm and reassuring, but the thing I appreciated most is that he didn't try to push me into anything. The other two doctors tried to talk me into more than I felt I needed. I didn't want to look twenty or thirty again. I just wanted to look the best I could at age fifty. The other doctors seemed more concerned about how much money they would make as opposed to what was the right thing for me.

Dr. Flaharty wanted what I wanted: to look like the best "me" I possibly could, without going overboard. In fact, he suggested it wasn't eyelid surgery that I needed, but rather a brow lift. He also suggested a mini-lift, which is not as extensive as a full face lift, but a procedure that would lift the bottom two thirds of my face and neck.

It was about six months from the time I started thinking about doing something until the time I finally scheduled the surgery. I take a long time to make big decisions, and this was a big decision. I told my daughter and my boyfriend about my upcoming surgery. My daughter was really excited for me. My boyfriend said the right thing: he told me I looked beautiful the way I was, but if it was what I wanted, to go for it. I also told a couple of my close friends. They were really excited, too, and couldn't wait to see the new me.

I'm a really positive person, so once I made up my mind, I knew it would turn out great. The day of the surgery I was a little nervous— after all, I was going under the knife—but mostly I was excited and I couldn't wait to see what I looked like after the procedure. My boyfriend took me to the surgery center and picked me up. Everyone at the surgery center was wonderful and reassuring. They really made it a breeze. I had no trepidation at all.

My total recovery time was around two weeks. Initially I was a bit sore…it was uncomfortable for a few days, but nothing I couldn't handle. In fact, I didn't even take the pain pills that were prescribed. I was teaching a couple of college classes at that time. I went back to work while I still had a little bit of bruising, but I was able to cover it up with makeup.

After my procedure, people's reactions were really interesting: my daughter was thrilled and thought I looked fabulous. Most people would look at me and ask if I had a new haircut. It was like they knew I did something, but they didn't know what. I feel like I look a lot younger now, even ten years later. People— especially women— actually ask me how old I am. Some people come right out and say, "You look great. Did you have some work done?" I can tell they're dying to know. If they ask, I tell them because I have nothing to hide. I'm really happy I had the surgery and feel fortunate I could afford it.

Now I go to Dr. Flaharty about once a year for fillers and a little Botox. I consider it my maintenance program. I also take great care of myself: I'm a tennis player, but I wear big sunglasses, a big hat, and lots of sunscreen. I use a good moisturizer, exercise, and drink lots of water. I want to stay young as long as I can.

My advice to others: if you're thinking about it, go for it. Interview several doctors and talk to a lot of people who've had work done. Find a doctor you're completely comfortable with. Don't scrimp on the price. If you can't afford to do it, just have fillers and Botox. Don't go to a hack surgeon who's going to ruin you.

One last thing…if you think it's going to change your life, it won't. There are women who keep going back and getting more and more procedures. If you're not happy inside, no plastic surgery is going to change that. It's not a magic pill that will cure all your problems. One of my daughter's friends keeps having surgery. She thinks the next procedure will be the one to make her feel better about herself. She's done everything and is still no happier than before. It can become an addiction. You think it's going to be a magic potion to cure everything.

FAT TRANSFER

Today, we understand that facial rejuvenation isn't just about fighting gravity. It's also very much about restoring volume. We must look at the face in three dimensions to best appreciate how we age and the best path to true rejuvenation. Fat transfer is a surgical technique using living fat cells from your body to restore lost volume in the face. Fat transfer offers a more permanent solution to the loss of volume in the face when compared to fillers. Because the fat comes from your own body, there is no risk of rejection. The most common areas to inject are cheeks, temples, brows, under the eyes, the jawline, lower cheeks, and the chin.

This series of photos shows how the youthful contours are reestablished after fat transfer. We see the patient before and after fat transfer, and then a photo of her college-aged daughter. Notice the mother's resemblance to her daughter in the "after photo."

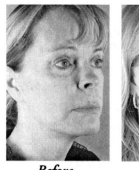 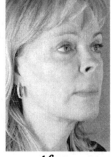 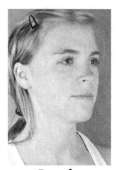

Before   *After*   *Daughter*

*This patient resembles her daughter after her youthful
fullness was restored with fat transfer.*

How Is It Done?

During your pre-op visit, you choose the area (belly, thighs, buttocks, arms) from which we will take the fat. Because we remove only a small amount of fat, the area from which the fat is taken will not derive much benefit. During the procedure, the fat is removed by liposuction. It is then purified to isolate the pure living fat cells before being delicately injected into selected areas on your face. It is an elegant procedure that requires only a few puncture wounds to harvest and replant the fat. We use a very specific technique when we inject the fat into your face, to ensure it develops a new blood supply. Not all the cells from the injected fat will survive. On average, 60–70 percent of the cells will remain long term.

How Long Does The Surgery Take?

The fat transfer procedure takes approximately two hours.

What is The Pain Factor?

You will have some mild soreness both at the donor site and the injection site.

Are There Any Side Effects?

There is some swelling and bruising which will last a few weeks.

What Is The Healing Process?

While the swelling and bruising can last a few weeks, you can resume your normal activities within a few days. We ask patients to be gentle with their face while cleansing and washing. As with all surgical procedures, we recommend light activity only for the first two weeks post-surgery. Full activity can be resumed after two weeks. Makeup can be worn a few days after the procedure if necessary.

How Long Before The Full Effect Is Realized?

The benefit of the fat transfer is seen immediately. Most of the swelling resolves in two weeks, but some additional swelling and fat loss will continue for 2–3 months. The final outcome is evident at three months.

How Long Does It Last?

We consider fat transfer permanent as the fat that survives will last for many years. Of course facial aging continues, (so future fat loss will occur,) but you are starting from a position of a much fuller face.

CHIN AUGMENTATION

When patients come in for a facial consultation, I always take a close look at their chin. Weakness of the chin can cause the face to be out of balance, weaken the jawline, and cause the neck to appear shorter and wider. For some people, a chin implant can balance the face, strengthen the jawline, and give the appearance of a longer, leaner, and more defined neck. When a patient complains of a weak chin—as was the case with Penore—I look at the chin in relation to the lips, nose, and anterior planes of the face, paying special attention to the projection of the nose and lips and how it compares to the projection of the chin from a side view. (You can read Penore's story in chapter twelve, *For Men Only*.)

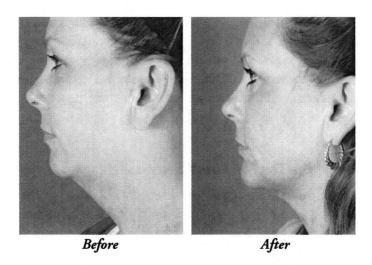

Before   *After*

The addition of a chin implant and neck liposuction
dramatically changes this patient's facial profile

How Is Chin Augmentation Done?

A small incision is made under the chin, where it will not be visible. A delicate pocket is developed over the jaw bone (anterior mandible) and the implant is placed into this custom designed pocket. The modern implants are made of soft silicone and conform perfectly to the contour of the jaw bone. These implants are soft and compressible. They blend well between the bone and muscle. The implant is delicately tapered and isn't visible or palpable after implantation. The small incision is closed with several layers of dissolvable sutures.

How Long Does The Surgery Take?

The chin augmentation procedure is a relatively brief procedure taking roughly forty-five minutes to complete.

What Is The Pain Factor?

There may be mild soreness during the first evening after your chin implant. Some degree of tenderness can last a few weeks.

Are There Any Side Effects?

Swelling, bruising, soreness, and numbness in the area of surgery are all possible, but are generally mild and resolve over a few weeks.

What Is The Healing Process?

The sutures under the chin are covered with a steri-strip. Patients put an ointment over the steri-strip for six days. All patients are placed on antibiotics to prevent infection. Although infections of chin implants are very rare, if infection does occur, the implant must be removed. Patients are asked to be gentle when washing the face for a few months to avoid moving the implant. The implant becomes encapsulated into place over a few months and then remains very stable.

How Long Before The Full Effect Is Realized?

The effect of a chin implant is seen immediately. Most of the swelling will resolve in a few weeks and final results are generally visible at one month..

CO_2 (CARBON DIOXIDE) LASER RESURFACING

Laser resurfacing with a carbon dioxide laser is for those patients with moderate to severe facial wrinkling who would not respond to the noninvasive skin lasers. The CO^2 laser is an ablative procedure, precisely removing the top layer of skin and then tightening the deeper layers by shrinking the collagen by as much as thirty percent. The results are truly amazing. Not only are all the brown sun spots removed in a single treatment, but 70–90 percent of the facial wrinkles are also eliminated.

How Is It Done?

As the laser is moved over the face, it emits pulses—or quick bursts—of energy to the skin surface. The CO_2 laser is highly absorbed by water, and the energy delivered to the skin will vaporize the epidermis (the surface layer of the skin.) Once the skin is cleaned, a second and third pass can be performed to tighten the dermal collagen, thus eliminating the wrinkles. The CO_2 laser is very accurate and can be adjusted for the patient's specific needs. Some patients may require only a light treatment with one pass of the laser, while others need up to three passes on stronger settings for the best results.

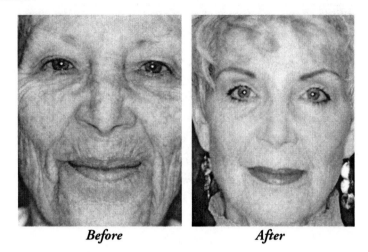

Before　　　　*After*

The CO_2 treatment can result in a dramatic improvement to severe sun damage and wrinkling

How Long Does It Take?

It takes approximately forty-five minutes to do the entire face.

What Is The Pain Factor?

An occlusive bandage is placed over the skin for the first 3–4 days. The bandage protects the skin and aids in quicker healing. There is mild discomfort for a few weeks; slight soreness, itching, burning, and sensitivity. This resolves slowly as the skin heals over the first few weeks.

Are There Any Side Effects?

It takes about two weeks for the new skin surface to heal after CO_2 laser resurfacing. During that time the patient will experience some itching and discomfort and require frequent ointments. The patient must stay out of the sun. The skin may stay pink or red (similar to a mild sunburn) for several months. Makeup can be used to camouflage the redness until it resolves.

What Is The Healing Process?

The post-procedure protocol for the CO_2 laser is a bit cumbersome. Following the procedure, a protective bandage—called Flexzan—with an opening for the eyes, nostrils and mouth is put over the entire face. This bandage remains in place for 3–4 days, at which point the patient comes back to the office to have the bandage removed. We recommend patients take a pain medication prior to having the bandage removed. After the bandage is removed the face is soaked to remove any dry, crusted areas. The face is then coated with ointment.

For the next ten days, the face is soaked with a vinegar and water solution two to three times per day. In between soaking the face, Vaseline or Aquaphor is applied to keep the skin moist. It is important to keep the face completely covered with one of these products in between soakings to keep the skin protected. A new layer of delicate pink skin will grow in approximately two weeks. Once the new skin has healed, facial cleansing is permitted using a gentle cleanser and an intensive moisturizer. We provide a kit that contains these two products plus sunscreen. Sun must be avoided for the two weeks following the procedure. In fact, we recommend that patients avoid excessive sun exposure for a few months after the procedure until the skin has normalized.

How Long Before The Full Effect Is Realized?

The full effect of the procedure is visible at one month, although it may take 2–6 months for all the pinkness to resolve. We offer a special makeup for our laser resurfacing patients and you can wear this makeup two weeks after your procedure.

DERMABRASION

Dermabrasion is a form of "surgical sanding" used to smooth out lines and wrinkles, especially around the mouth. Patients often confuse *dermabrasion* with *microdermabrasion*, but they are not the same. Microdermabrasion is a skin treatment—performed by a medical aesthetician—that removes dead cells from the surface of the skin and activates new collagen formation. Dermabrasion is a surgical procedure—performed by a doctor—that "abrades" the skin to reduce moderate to deep wrinkles, especially on the upper lip, corners of the mouth, lower lip, and chin area. Surgical dermabrasion is often combined with CO_2 laser resurfacing to rejuvenate the entire face, and can be more effective than CO_2 laser resurfacing for the tougher wrinkles around the mouth. Surgical dermabrasion is appropriate for moderate to heavy wrinkles in thick-skinned areas like the mouth. It is not appropriate for mild wrinkles or in thin-skinned areas like the eyelids.

How Is It Done?

Surgical dermabrasion involves using a spinning burr that accurately shaves off the superficial layers of the skin. Static wrinkles, or permanent wrinkles, are actually folds or "hills and valleys" within the skin. Surgical dermabrasion evens out those hills and valleys, reducing or eliminating the wrinkle.

How Long Does It Take?

It takes approximately 15–30 minutes to treat the areas around the mouth.

What Is The Pain Factor?

There is mild discomfort, redness, and sensitivity. This resolves as the skin heals.

Are There Any Side Effects?

The new skin will be pink for several weeks and can sometimes be slightly lighter in color (hypopigmented) once it heals completely due to the loss of pigment-making cells. Makeup can be used to camouflage the redness until it resolves.

What Is The Healing Process?

It takes 7–10 days for the new skin surface to heal after dermabrasion. (Similar to the CO_2 laser, the surface of the skin is removed and the new skin replaces the old.) During that time, the patient will experience redness and sensitivity. Ointment is applied several times a day. The healing process for dermabrasion is quicker than with the CO_2 laser. Sun must be avoided for the two weeks following the procedure. In fact, we recommend patients avoid excessive sun exposure for a few months after the procedure until the skin has normalized.

How Long Before The Full Effect Is Realized?

The full effect of the procedure is visible at two weeks, although it may take two months for all the pinkness to resolve. We offer a special makeup for our laser resurfacing patients; the makeup can be worn two weeks after the procedure.

PANFACIAL REJUVENATION AND THE HARMONIOUS LIFT

Every patient wants the best and most natural results with the least amount of surgery. The reality is that our faces tend to age globally and the most complete and natural facial rejuvenation is often achieved by doing a panfacial rejuvenation, which means doing every part of the face at once.

There are many advantages to this approach including *one* procedure and *one* recovery period, not to mention the stunning harmonious result when every part of the face is rejuvenated and nothing is left "undone." Imagine someone having a beautiful surgical rejuvenation of the face—everything *except* the bags under their eyes. After surgery, what do you think would be the very first thing that person would see when looking in the mirror? It wouldn't be the beautiful result; it would be the bags under their eyes. (Think about redecorating an entire room, but leaving one raggedy old chair.) If a beautiful rejuvenation is done on the face, but one area is left untouched, the result can be attention-getting…but it's not the kind of attention you want.

The right mix of procedures is different for everyone and may entail one or more of the following: a brow lift, eyelid surgery, face and neck lift, fat transfer, neck liposuction, fillers, and Botox. Whatever is the specific formula for you, it makes sense to address it all at once. Not only will you have a much better result, but you'll have a more natural and longer-lasting result. Panfacial rejuvenation isn't right or necessary for everyone, but when the analysis dictates a more comprehensive approach, it is certainly the most powerful rejuvenation technique available. What's more is that combining these multiple procedures saves money: since everything is done at once, the patient's cost for the operating room and anesthesia (which is added to the doctor's fee) is a one-time cost. And…when multiple procedures are done at one time, there is no additional downtime; it's still roughly two weeks. What's more impressive than Ruthann's panfacial rejuvenation photos is her tenacious spirit as a single woman who came to see us for the first time when she was approaching age fifty.

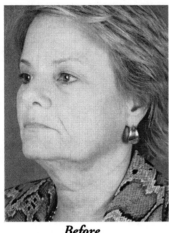 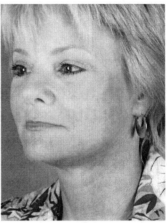

Before   *After*

Panfacial rejuvenation is a comprehensive approach to facial lifting: all aspects of the aging face are addressed at once for a complete and harmonious transformation.

It Took Me Ten Years to Do it, But It Was Worth Every Penny

Ruthann

Age: 57

When I turned forty, I didn't like what I saw in the mirror: I had developed a double chin and my eyelids were drooping so you couldn't even see my eye shadow. That's when I started thinking about doing something. I went for a consult with a plastic surgeon and he showed me on a computer what I would look like if I had some work done. I would look gorgeous! But… it was totally out of my budget.

Ten years went by and I never stopped thinking about having a face lift. I was a single woman approaching fifty. I hated my neck, so I wore turtle necks a lot, but then my double-chin would sit on top of the turtle neck. It really bothered me and made me feel old. Finally, getting a face lift was in my budget. I sold my house, made some extra money, and decided to use that money on me. I did a lot of research on plastic surgeons in the area. I asked for referrals and did a lot of research online. I didn't take this lightly at all. I made appointments and went for consultations with four doctors. I had made up my mind that I wasn't shopping for the best price, but rather the doctor who had the best reputation and with whom I felt most comfortable. I chose Dr. Flaharty because he's very specialized in that he does only faces. He didn't overpromise. I asked him how long my face lift would last. He said, "The minute you walk out after surgery, you will start aging." I loved his honesty. I also felt really good about his staff. We decided I would have a face lift, brow lift, and my upper and lower eyelids done.

Once I decided on Dr. Flaharty, it took about two months before I had the surgery. I had to wait for the sale of my house to go through. Here in Florida, my business is a lot less busy in the summer and I wanted to wait for the slow season.

I was so excited! I told everyone I knew that I was getting a face lift. I had to take time off from work and I didn't feel like I needed to hide anything. A lot of people didn't understand why I was doing it. Honestly, I think they were jealous. Getting a face lift is a very personal thing and everyone has their own reasons for doing it. It wasn't important to me that some people didn't understand. I was doing it and I wasn't looking for approval. If anyone wanted to join in on my excitement, that was great. I didn't tell people because I needed reassurance. I told them because I was excited.

The morning of the surgery I was all wound up: I had waited years for this. I had been up all night. I had followed all my instructions: I ate the right things. I didn't eat any of the foods that make you swell and I didn't drink. I flew my sister here to take care of me for the week. Everything was ready.

I remember thinking to myself that I was prepared for whatever pain I would have. I didn't matter. It would be so worth it. But there really was no pain. The first night I had a bad headache and that was the worst of it. After three days, I felt really great and on the fourth day, I was myself again. I went back to work after two weeks. I had no bruises. No one would ever know I had anything done. Everyone told me I looked great.

The week before my surgery, I had met a man ten years younger than I. It just so happened he was going out of town for a month. It was perfect timing. I told him I was having some work done, that I hated my saggy jaw and neck, and the next time he saw me, they would be gone. When he came back, he didn't think I looked a lot different. Of course, he hadn't noticed that you couldn't see my eye shadow before. We've now been living together for six years.

My advice to others: it's worth every penny. It will change how you feel about yourself. It will make you happier. Of course, if you're not a happy person to begin with, it's not going to help. It will make you look better, but it won't fix your problems. It will make you take better care of your health...you will look younger and you will respect your heath more. Research your doctor big time. Remember, it's not about the price. It's about your doctor's reputation. A doctor has to earn his reputation. Each of the four doctors I saw was top-notch. For me, Dr. Flaharty was the best because at the time he was the only doctor who did faces only.

A FINAL NOTE ON SURGERY

Although surgical rejuvenation of the face is the gold standard in terms of long-lasting rejuvenation, it does not stop the continual, inevitable aging process. The positive changes made through surgery are long lasting. However, the inevitable aging process will result in ongoing and progressive changes to the face over time. We cannot reasonably expect the effects to last forever. In truth, the concerns that are taken care of with surgery are taken care of for years, but aging—and the changes that come with it—will continue. Future treatment can be designed to address these new changes.

TWELVE

· · · · · · · · · · · · · ·

FOR MEN ONLY

A guy's guide to facial rejuvenation

While men are still in the minority when it comes to facial rejuvenation, the number of men seeking cosmetic procedures is growing at a fast pace. Men currently represent about ten percent of the patients in our practice. The number of male patients continues to grow. When I started my practice more than twenty years ago, it was a rare sight to see a man in our waiting room. Today, no one blinks an eye at the sight of a man.

Men tend to be less diligent than women when it comes to wearing sunscreen. The outdoor lifestyle we enjoy here in Southwest Florida, combined with the more than 150 golf courses in our area, are the causes of a lot of sun-damaged facial skin for men. It's no secret that a large part of our population here in Southwest Florida is baby boomers and retirees. We see many male boomers and part-time retirees who still want to work, yet feel the pressure to look younger as they compete in the job market. We also see men who are trying to "keep pace" with their wives who are more likely to avail themselves of cosmetic enhancements.

Here's the story of one of our baby boomer male patients, Penore.

I Looked in the Mirror and Saw...My Father!

Penore

Age: 62

About four years ago, I looked in the mirror one day and was startled: I was becoming my Dad. I didn't act like him, I didn't dress like him, but I looked like him. My Dad was an old man at age fifty. Here I was, nearing sixty, and I certainly didn't feel like an old man, but I was starting to look like one. As I thought about it, I felt people were starting to treat me differently: they were treating me as if I were an old man. I guess that's what spurred me to start checking out doctors and considering plastic surgery. I never would have guessed I'd have done this.

I started checking out all the doctors in the area; I'm a serious comparative shopper. I looked at numerous plastic surgeons and went to a total of three for consultations. When I went to Dr. Flaharty, I just knew. I was impressed with the professionalism and the calming ambience of his office. The level of professionalism was something I just didn't see in the other offices. Dr. Flaharty was very personable and took all the time necessary. I liked his attitude. I liked what he said. I felt he spoke to me like a person, not as a potential patient. He never tried to sell me, and in fact, he told me "no" on a couple of things. Initially I thought to myself, "I'll go somewhere else and get what I want," but then I realized that I had come to completely trust him and he is the expert, not me. He addressed my wants, but he expressed his opinion and stated it was his opinion.

When I went to Dr. Flaharty, it was for a consultation on looking better, not necessarily a consultation for a face lift. I was thinking, "Maybe a minor tuck here or there." Initially I had thought about the Lifestyle Lift because I had seen it on TV, but then when I did my research, I knew it wasn't for me. I mentioned the Lifestyle Lift to Dr. Flaharty. He was so good about explaining it. He never put it down, but he explained what I could expect from a Lifestyle Lift. I also had in mind the possibility of a chin implant as I always felt I had a weak jaw as opposed to a rugged, masculine jaw. Dr. Flaharty's opinion was that I didn't need a chin implant. Instead, he suggested a mandible on either side of the chin which broadened my chin. (That's one of the things I did and I love the way it looks.) Dr. Flaharty understood that

I didn't want to look 30 years younger…I just wanted to look better.

I ended up getting a face lift, a neck lift, and the mandible on either side of the chin. The neck makes all the difference in the world. I see all these people who've had work done to their face, and that beautiful new face is sitting on this turkey neck. I just think, "It just doesn't look right." I don't have the neck I had when I was twenty or thirty, but I can say I don't have as bad a neck as I had when I was forty.

The procedure itself was handled in the most professional way. The surgery center is just fabulous. Surgery is surgery, and anyone will have some butterflies, but they immediately put you at ease. You're spoken to four or five times to be sure everyone is on exactly the same page. I took one week out of work and went back three-quarter time after the week. At that point, the stitches were out and I had just a little bit of pinkness around the ears; the bruising was almost completely gone. I was back to myself in terms of energy.

I think the days of being totally secretive (and embarrassed) about getting plastic surgery are gone. I give Joan Rivers a lot of the credit for that. She looks a little plastic, I admit, but she looks beautiful, and especially for her age. The idea of a man getting plastic surgery may be a little taboo, but I have to sell myself every day. If I have a chance to make my business look better, to upgrade my business, I do it. I'm my best sales person and I have to look the part. I shared with a number of clients that I was getting some plastic surgery and the reaction was amazingly positive. Once I told some of my clients, they admitted to having had some work done themselves. In fact, they seemed delighted to give me tips on how to get ready for the surgery and what to do after.

I could not be any happier with the result. I'm in the public and see clients every day. Everyone tells me "you look so good." Unless I choose to tell them, nobody guesses I had any work done. I look so rested, refreshed. I get mistaken all the time for being in my forties. No one guesses – ever – that I'm in my sixties. I don't think I'm any different from anyone else: we all want to look the best we can. It's funny, because people know something's different. I'm often asked if I got my eyes done and I can truthfully say, "No, I didn't!" I get fillers occasionally now. We always think of pulling the face to get rid of wrinkles and look younger, but the aging process is a lot about hollowing and that needs to be addressed. The fillers are so minimally invasive. There's no downtime.

That day you have a bit of red where the injections are, but that's it.

My advice to others: do your homework and check out the doctors. Check references. It's a big decision. Ask yourself, "What would I be able to do if I looked better than I look right now?" Our face is our window to the world and it's the first thing people see and we want it to be the best it can be, so why not go for it? When you look better, you feel better. It gives you a new confidence. Everything about the business world today is confidence and youth. You don't want to look too young, but you don't want to look like an old fogy.

Penore is among the increasing number of men who want to look younger and are willing to do something about it. In 2011, men in the United States underwent more than 1.1 million cosmetic procedures, including both minimally invasive and surgical procedures.[11]

MEN ARE FROM MARS

It sounds a bit silly to mention the obvious: men are different from women. But in the world of facial rejuvenation, those differences mean there are distinct contrasts in the approach to facial rejuvenation when it comes to men as compared to women. Skin thickness, hair pattern, bone structure, and the soft tissues of the face (muscle and fat) are different for men and women, and must be taken into account when planning facial rejuvenation for a man. Men tend to have rectangular faces with prominent brow bones and jawlines, as compared to women who generally have softer, more oval faces. Another major difference is that women naturally have arched eyebrows; men do not. Men have lower, flatter eyebrows than women. All of these gender-specific features must be understood, taken into consideration, and preserved to achieve the best and most natural result for men.

SKIN CARE

We have a number of male patients who get facials and use our skin care products. As we discussed in chapter five, good skin care need not be complicated or cost a fortune. Taking into consideration each individual's skin, our medical aesthetician recommends a simple, yet effective skin care routine. We do not believe in fancy product packaging, so men, you won't be accused of using products made for women.

LASER HAIR REMOVAL

Laser hair removal has become an increasingly popular solution in recent years for men who are looking to reduce excessive or unwanted hair. Laser hair removal can be done anywhere on the body, but the most popular areas for men are ears and backs. About twenty percent of our laser hair removal patients are men. As we discussed in chapter nine, this procedure uses a low energy laser to permanently reduce unwanted hair in a safe, effective, quick manner.

BOTULINIUM TOXIN TYPE A AND FILLERS

In 2011, Botulinium Toxin Type A (Botox and Dysport) topped the list of minimally invasive procedures for men, with 5.6 million procedures performed, while men enjoyed 1.8 million injections of fillers.[12] Once again, knowledge of the male facial anatomy and experience in injecting both neurotoxins and fillers is key to a successful outcome. Most men do not want an arched brow, which can be achieved with Botox, but instead they just want their forehead wrinkles removed.

UPPER AND LOWER EYELID SURGERY

Both upper and lower eyelid surgery are popular procedures for men. The upper eyelid lift corrects heavy, hooded eyelids, while lower eyelid surgery takes care of wrinkles and bags under the eyes. We've all seen male movie stars or television personalities who've had bad face lifts. If you look closely, often you'll see the eyebrows have been unnaturally arched. Other times, the problem is too much surgery, resulting in an unnatural, hollow look. This can be avoided with attention to detail and good technique.

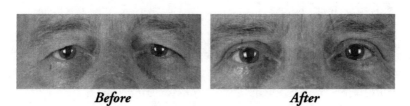

Before   *After*

This gentleman had upper eyelid surgery.

BROW LIFT

Brow lifts are less common for men and should be much more subtle than in women. A male brow pattern is lower and heavier. Men often look quite natural with a slightly heavy brow. When brow lifts are performed on men, the normal, flat shape of the male brow needs to be preserved. The arched pattern of the female brow must be avoided at all costs when performing brow lifts on men.

CHIN AUGMENTATION

Like Penore, men are often concerned with a weak chin. Some men wear a goatee to cover up a weak chin. As surgery goes, the chin augmentation is a rather simple procedure—taking only around forty-five minutes—with very little downtime. (Refer to chapter eleven for more details on chin augmentation.)

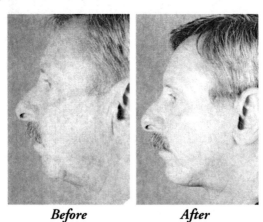

Before   *After*

The addition of a chin implant improves this patient's jawline and facial balance.

FACE AND NECK LIFT

The biggest area of growth in our practice regarding cosmetic surgery for men is the number of men requesting lower face and neck lifts. Men are taking better care of themselves, staying healthier and living longer. They are also staying more socially active and working longer. Many men are bothered by the loose skin in the neck and to a lesser extent, the jowls. This loose neck skin can be accentuated for men who wear a shirt and tie to work. A lower face and neck lift can really clean up the jaw line and neck line, restoring confidence in men as they age. In the past year, I've had many men in their seventies and eighties come to the office to discuss face and neck lift procedures. These procedures are becoming much more common in a population of patients once considered "too old" for surgery. Times are a-changing.

THE BOTTOM LINE FOR MEN

The bottom line for men and facial rejuvenation is this: our society places a great deal of value on looking young and fresh. Today, men of all ages and all walks of life are visiting my practice wanting a more youthful appearance—and for good reason. Men are living healthier, more active lifestyles than ever before and that translates to holding themselves to the same high physical standards in the workplace—and the culture. It's not uncommon for us to hear from male patients in their sixties that they're the oldest guy in the office, and are getting passed over on opportunities by someone fifteen years younger. More and more, older men are looking at threats from their younger, technology-savvy colleagues and they're doing everything they can to remain current. As retirement age continues to rise, it isn't uncommon for men to come in for a procedure or two, and then become regular skin care and facial clients. Regardless of the reasons why they choose facial rejuvenation, we find that our male patients are exceedingly pleased with the ease of the experience and astonished by the results.

THIRTEEN
· · · · · · · · · · · · · · · · ·

Postscript on Pricing

"How much does it **cost?**" is one of the most frequently-asked questions when patients come to the office for a consultation, and we answer that question in detail. In our office, the pricing discussion takes place with our Patient Care Coordinator. My examination and consultation with the patient generates a list of potential treatments—a "roadmap to rejuvenation" so to speak—including both surgical and nonsurgical options. Our Patient Care Coordinator then reviews pricing with the patient: the specific costs for each procedure are discussed, including the additional fees for anesthesia and the facility, if surgery is contemplated. The "roadmap" is used as a guide for the pricing discussion. Procedures can be staged to match the interest and budget of the patient.

Fees for facial cosmetic surgery vary widely in different areas of the country and from practitioner to practitioner. Fees are higher in areas with a higher cost of living, such as New York and California. The cost of practicing medicine is more expensive in these areas and these costs are passed on to you, the consumer. Within the same area, fees for a given procedure can vary from physician to physician based on experience and practice style. A "specialist" who focuses on a specific procedure may charge more than a doctor who offers a wide range of procedures, but hasn't developed a unique expertise in one area. Experience is also a factor. Physicians who have developed exceptional skills by focusing on a specific area over many years will likely charge more than a physician just getting started out of training. Believe it or not, the price of a face lift can vary from $5,000 to $50,000 based on these factors. Below are some pricing guidelines—based on our practice—for the common facial cosmetic procedures we've discussed throughout this book.

We are fortunate in Southwest Florida to be a destination area with beautiful weather and modest prices. Patients come here from around the country, and around the globe, to receive top-quality medical care at reasonable prices. And what's even better is that they can relax and recover in this tropical hideaway and return home looking refreshed.

SKIN CARE

Skin care is the least expensive entry point for facial cosmetic enhancement. Skin care procedures—including therapeutic facials, microdermabrasion, micropeels, and light laser peels—can range from $100–$250. At our office, you can get a full array of skin care products for $100–$200 and these will last at least 3–4 months.

BOTOX AND FILLERS

Botox treatments range from $300–$1,000 and fillers from $500–$2,500 per treatment. Botox and fillers are often combined into a single treatment session (the Liquid face lift.) The cost for the Liquid Face Lift is the sum of the cost of all the products. To make things more interesting, some physicians charge for neurotoxins by the area (forehead, between the eyes and crow's feet, etc.,) and some charge by the unit. We have opted to treat by the area, and we are happy to see patients back in the office within a few weeks to give them more product—if they need it—at no additional charge. Neurotoxins are fast becoming a commodity with many physician specialties performing injections. We believe that the expertise in performing the injections is paramount to achieving a good result; we stand behind our work, preferring to charge for a result rather than an amount delivered.

LASERS AND ULTHERAPY

Office-based lasers including the IPL and fractional lasers range from $500–$700 per treatment with a full series running about $2,100. Ultherapy costs $1,800–$3,500 per treatment depending on the areas treated (upper face, lower face, full face.)

SURGERY

Surgical procedures can range from $3,000 for an upper eyelid surgery to $30,000 for a complete rejuvenation of the face, which may include a brow lift, face and neck lift, neck liposuction, eyelid surgery, fat transfer, Botox, fillers, and skin treatments.

A FINAL WORD ON PRICE

The old adage "you get what you pay for" rings true in all aspects of facial rejuvenation. Over the years, we've seen many patients who have gone to fly-by-night operations or "surgery mills" to save money. The results are usually telling. Visible scars, distorted features, unnatural contours, and incomplete results are the hallmark of poor work and these problems can be difficult—if not impossible—to fix. We can design a plan which makes sense for your budget, even if that means doing a little bit at a time. When it comes to your face, please don't cut corners.

FOURTEEN

. . . .

Conclusion

As a cosmetic surgeon, my work is as intrinsically rewarding for me on the inside as it is for a patient on the outside. And that said, we rarely encounter a patient who doesn't say that the rewards of facial rejuvenation are more satisfying for them internally than externally. Aging is a part of the natural process of life and as human beings, we have to love what's on the inside as much as what our faces or bodies show on the outside. That is the *true* beauty of what my patients—male and female—and I do together. What begins as a feeling of unease with what we see in the mirror becomes a peacefulness within. When the face is brought into alignment with how the mind feels, one has an all-around sense of well-being and self-confidence. To you, my patients, and to all of you who may come to join our family at Azul, thanks for inspiring us with your timeless beauty—both inside and out.

ACKNOWLEDGEMENTS

I would first like to thank my mother and father for their unconditional love and support during my formative years of education and development. My father was a physician who loved his patients and the science of medicine. He was my first and most powerful role model, and the reason I chose to pursue a career in medicine.

I would like to thank Dr. Joseph Flanagan, who played a major role in my decision to pursue Oculoplastic Surgery as a discipline. Joe's boundless energy has always been infectious. Dr. Richard Anderson, my preceptor and mentor in the field of Oculofacial Plastic Surgery, has continued to inspire me with his enthusiasm, insights and unwavering support. Rick is a world-class surgeon, scholar and friend. He provided the foundation for my career.

I would like to thank my staff for their unwavering commitment to excellence and compassion. They are always willing to go the extra mile to make our patients comfortable and well cared for.

To my patients, I would say that you are by far the greatest teachers. I learn from each and every one of you and appreciate your faith in me as your doctor.

Lastly, I would like to thank my wife and children. Kristen, a career woman herself, understands the commitment of time and energy required for a life in medicine, and has always been supportive of my efforts—even when she was the one to make sacrifices. And to my beautiful girls, Katie, Caroline and Kendall: I love you all so much. Thank you for helping me to keep it all in perspective.

An Invitation For Our Readers

You're invited to visit *www.AzulBeauty.com/readers-only* for a complimentary gift from Dr. Flaharty.

Endnotes

1 American Society for Aesthetic Plastic Surgery. Quoted with permission.

2 Study conducted by Howard N. Langstein, M.D., Professor and Chief of Plastic and Reconstructive Surgery, University of Rochester Medical Center. Quoted with permission.

3 Florida Board of Medicine.

4 Milady Publishing Corporation. 1998. Milady's Standard Textbook for Professional Aestheticians by Joel Gerson.

5 As told in Rosie and Mrs. America: Perceptions of Women in the 1930s and 1940s (Images and Issues of Women in the Twentieth Century), Catherine Gourley, Twenty-First Century Books, September 1, 2007.

6 Basal-cell carcinoma, a form of skin cancer, is the most common form of cancer. It is rarely life-threatening and rarely metastasizes. http://en.wikipedia.org/wiki/Basal-cell_carcinoma.

7 Mohs surgery is microscopically controlled surgery used to treat common types of skin cancer. http://en.wikipedia.org/wiki/Mohs_surgery.

8 American Society of Plastic Surgeons. Quoted with permission.

9 American Society of Plastic Surgeons. Quoted with permission.

10 American Society of Plastic Surgeons. Quoted with permission.

11 American Society of Plastic Surgeons. Quoted with permission.

12 American Society of Plastic Surgeons. Quoted with permission. Botulinum Toxin Type A numbers are based on the number of sites injected.

CPSIA information can be obtained at www.ICGtesting.com
Printed in the USA
LVOW121807020513

332035LV00016B/943/P